S0-BPY-696

AACN organization and management of critical-care facilities

AACN organization and management of critical-care facilities

Edited by

DIANE C. ADLER, R.N., M.A., CCRN

Clinical Nurse Specialist in Critical Care,
Emergency Medical Service System;
Past President, American Association of Critical-Care Nurses,
New York, New York

NORMA J. SHOEMAKER, R.N., M.N.

Executive Director,
Society of Critical Care Medicine,
Anaheim, California

with **32** illustrations

RA975.5
I56
A15
1979

The C. V. Mosby Company

ST. LOUIS · TORONTO · LONDON   1979

350826

Copyright © 1979 by The C. V. Mosby Company

All rights reserved. No part of this book may be reproduced in any manner without written permission of the publisher.

Printed in the United States of America

The C. V. Mosby Company
11830 Westline Industrial Drive, St. Louis, Missouri 63141

Library of Congress Cataloging in Publication Data

Main entry under title:

AACN organization and management of critical-care
    facilities.

    Bibliography: p.
    Includes index.
    1. Intensive care units.   2. Intensive care nursing.
3. Critical care medicine.   I. Adler, Diane C.
II. Shoemaker, Norma J.   III. American Association of
Critical-Care Nurses. [DNLM: 1. Critical care—Organization
and administration.   2. Intensive care units—Organization
and administration. WX218 A104]
RA975.5.I56A15   362.1   78-31498
ISBN 0-8016-0130-4

C/CB/B   9   8   7   6   5   4   3   2   1   01/A/011

Contributors

Christopher W. Bryan-Brown, M.D., F.A.C.A., F.C.C.P.

Director, Surgical-Respiratory Intensive Care Unit,
The Mount Sinai Medical Center,
New York, New York

Neil M. Goodwin, F.F.A.R.C.S.

Principal Specialist in charge of Intensive Care Units,
Addington and King Edward VIII Hospitals,
Durban, South Africa

Dennis M. Greenbaum, M.D., F.A.C.P.

Chief, Medical Intensive Care Unit,
St. Vincent's Hospital and Medical Center of New York,
New York, New York

Jane M. Kahn, R.N., M.N.

President, Critical Care Services, Inc.,
Los Angeles, California

Kateri Heckathorn, R.N., M.N.S.A.

Chairman, Intensive Care Nursing Service,
Massachusetts General Hospital,
Boston, Massachusetts

Kathryn M. Lewis, R.N., CCRN, M.Ed.

Instructor, Critical Care Clinical Service,
Good Samaritan Hospital,
Phoenix, Arizona

Leslie K. Sampson, R.N., CCRN

Patient Care Coordinator, Intensive Care Unit, Emergency Unit,
and Recovery Room,
Albert Einstein Medical Center, Northern Division,
Philadelphia, Pennsylvania

William C. Shoemaker, M.D., F.A.C.S.

Professor, Department of Surgery,
University of California, Los Angeles;
Chief, Acute Care Center,
Harbor/UCLA Medical Center,
Torrance, California

Sharon A. Smith, R.N., M.S.

Special Projects Director,
Massachusetts General Hospital,
Boston, Massachusetts

Warren F. Stevens, Ph.D.

Former Executive Director,
American Association of Critical-Care Nurses,
Irvine, California

Judith Thams, M.S.

Registered Professional Industrial Engineer;
Director of Planning and Research,
Anaheim Memorial Hospital,
Anaheim, California

James A. Van Drimmelen, B.A.

Architect; President, Facilities Planning,
Rolling Bay, Washington

Sharyl Justham Verillo, R.N., B.A.

Director of In-service Education,
Bay Harbor Hospital,
Harbor City, California

To the teams we've worked with. . . .

Foreword

It is a pleasure to introduce a book edited by two persons for whom I have such great admiration. Their recommendations are based on extensive knowledge of critical-care problems and wide experience in this important and expanding field.

In commenting on the book, I want to record a page of history that should be remembered. The poliomyelitis respirator centers of the 1950s were an early version of present-day critical-care facilities. They provided a high level of care not previously available. Perhaps for the first time, the respirator centers systematically gathered together a great diversity of specialties to combat a complex and baffling disease. Besides treatment, they were dedicated to research, demonstration, and teaching. A major element in their success was the education and training that evolved into superlative nursing and medical practice. The centers brought educators and practitioners together, so that consummate skills were developed and passed along to an ever-widening circle.

Before 1950, polio patients were scattered throughout the country, some of them isolated in iron lungs, in large or small hospitals. When new epidemics occurred, they often struck communities that had not seen polio for years, so that physicians and nurses were unprepared to cope with the special problems that suddenly confronted them.

The medical director of the National Foundation for Infantile Paralysis at this time was Dr. Kenneth S. Landauer. He has told me that Dr. James L. Wilson of Boston Children's Hospital first suggested that these scattered patients be moved to centers for intensive care by specialists. Landauer reasoned that such grouping would permit far better treatment—at much less cost. New ideas could be tried and evaluated promptly, and when successful, passed on quickly to other centers, and from them to neighboring hospitals. The grouping of patients facilitated research studies. It built up morale and hope and produced other benefits.

Modern critical-care facilities fill a different role of course. But like their earlier counterparts, they combine a wide range of disciplines with a superior level of nursing and medical practice. Using new technologies in support of established principles, the staff of these units now save patients whose multiple problems would otherwise be overwhelming. Modern critical-care facilities are a step into the widening future of health care.

John Haven Emerson
Cambridge, Massachusetts

Preface

As early as 1863 Florence Nightingale noted that "It is not uncommon, in small country hospitals, to have a recess or small room leading from the operating theatre in which the patients remain until they have recovered, or at least recovered from the immediate effects of the operation."[1]

From the beginning of organized nursing Florence Nightingale recognized that nurses provided better care when the sickest patients were closest to the nursing station. The remaining patients were then distributed away from the nursing station with the least ill located farthest from the source of care. This attempt to categorize and systematize the patient care requirements was an early form of intensive and progressive care and was used widely through the era of the large open wards. Prior to the advent of recovery rooms and intensive care units, it was essential that such a system be used to ensure the safety of the patients.

Although many hospitals probably did use this method, it was in 1923 that Johns Hopkins Hospital reported the establishment of a three-bed unit, specifically for the intensive care of neurosurgical patients.[2]

By 1930, Dr. M. Kirschner of the University of Tübingen's surgical hospital in Germany identified the need for a special department to care for critically ill patients as well as those recovering from surgery.[3] Kirschner's idea was to concentrate the most skilled nurses with an experienced physician/ director responsible for the coordination of patient care. Kirschner believed that this method would improve care.[4] That belief has survived the test of time, and is the concept on which present intensive care units are organized.

With the rapid expansion of special surgical techniques, during the following decades, more sophisticated postoperative care was required. Without this postoperative care even the best surgical skills left the patient's life in jeopardy. If unconscious or barely responsive patients were returned to the general floors to be recovered by nurses with many other responsibilities, one might question the value of surgery when the patient's life was inadequately protected after leaving the operating room.

The anesthesiologist and surgeon realized it was no longer possible for them to remain with the patient throughout the postanesthesia recovery period. Both nurses and physicians recognized the danger to patients' well-being and began discussing alternatives.

An interim solution was to confiscate any available space that could be converted for the concentrated care of these postanesthesia patients. This practice evolved into the present-day postanesthesia recovery areas. The recovery room concept was not carefully thought out and planned, but developed in response to an immediate and urgent need. This also holds true for the development of most other critical-care areas. The early days of critical care were, in fact, intensive nursing care units. The sickest patients were concentrated closest to the source of care, the nurses.

During World War II the need for recovery rooms increased rapidly because of the large number of casualties requiring stabilization and/or surgery and aftercare and also because of the limited numbers of available nurses.[5] The nursing shortage was also felt in the United States, spurring the development of recovery rooms at home as well as in the war zones.[6]

Then in the 1950s, after years of laboratory experimentation, cardiac surgery came to fruition. The word spread rapidly, and persons with congenital and acquired heart defects flocked to the medical centers that could provide this surgical intervention. In spite of the risk these surgical procedures carried, persons came from all over the world seeking relief and an improved quality of life. Those from South America and Europe came by sea because they could not tolerate the variable airline cabin pressures. Others traveled with oxygen cylinders as their constant companions.

Surgical skills were available, patients were arriving pleading for help, and nurses and physicians were struggling to justify the necessity of an appropriately staffed intensive care area for these cardiac surgical patients.

Establishing a core of full-time nurses with special preparation in the care of cardiac surgical patients became mandatory. It was recognized early that the patient's prognosis correlated with the nurse's skill and experience.[4] Yet, in attempting to establish a core of full-time nurses, oftentimes bitter political battles ensued.

The physicians and nurses involved banded together, determined to provide necessary care in spite of what seemed to be insurmountable obstacles. Thus, these teams developed out of necessity just as had the early recovery rooms. The nurses and physicians knew that unless they were able to work together as a team, their mutual goal of patient survival would never be achieved. It became obvious that the physician and nurse could no longer work in a master-servant relationship. The development of a reciprocal collegial relationship was mandatory and eventually succeeded among these team members. Enhanced by the pioneering spirit in knowing they were on the brink of many important discoveries, these teams persevered. An internal support system developed that provided the team with confidence and the peer support to tackle any problem in the interest of providing the patient care required. What was lacking in facilities, equipment, financial support, and only partially understood postoperative techniques was compensated for by constant surveillance and tender loving care of every patient.

These nurse-physician teams functioned autonomously. The contract was a moral one between the patient and the team and the team members themselves. Few people outside the immediate area understood or appreciated what these teams were attempting to accomplish. Since little communication existed between the administration and these teams, there was likewise minimal accountability.

Today, remnants of this team isolation can still be seen. More frequently, as the advantages of intensive care teams are demonstrated, communication with the outside world improves.

Just as the team identity, spirit, and effort made possible the progress of the 1950s, the future depends on the continuation, strengthening, and development of the team concept. That is what this book is all about.

Diane C. Adler
Norma J. Shoemaker

REFERENCES

1. Nightingale, F.: Notes on hospitals, ed. 3, Essex, England, 1863, Longman, Green, Longman, Roberts & Green.
2. Harvey, A. M.: Neurosurgical genius—Walter Edward Dandy, Johns Hopkins Med. J. **135:**358-368, 1974.
3. Kirschner, M.: Zum Neubau der Chirurgischen Universitätsklinik Tübingen, Der Chirurg **2:**54-61, 1930.
4. Hilberman, M.: The evolution of intensive care units, Crit. Care Med. 3(4):159-165, 1975.
5. Dunn, F. E., and Shupp, M. G.: The recovery room: a wartime economy, Am. J. Nurs. 43:279-281, 1943.
6. Conboy, C. E.: A recovery room, Am. J. Nurs. 47:686-687, 1947.

Contents

SECTION FIVE   **CONSIDERATIONS FOR PATIENT CARE**

12   **Monitoring the critically ill patient,** 175

William C. Shoemaker

13   **Data collection,** 188

Dennis M. Greenbaum

FORMATION STAGES

The formation, or idea phase, that may culminate in the construction of a critical-care unit is the result of one of the following circumstances: a new hospital facility is to be constructed, an existing hospital does not have a critical-care unit, or replacement is required for an existing unit. If an intensive care unit (ICU) is to be built to replace or supplement an existing unit, it is generally because the present structure is overused, inadequate, or outmoded. The persons who initially identify the need for a critical-care unit then proceed to collect the data necessary to support their position. A written presentation of the supporting facts and figures should be presented to the appropriate committees for consideration. Warren F. Stevens discusses the many steps involved in bringing a critical-care unit to fruition (Chapter 1). He places particular emphasis on documenting actual need for the additional service in the community rather than construction for construction's sake. The so-called edifice complex should be a thing of the past!

To the uninitiated, the requirements of various agencies may be overwhelming, and frustration is a normal response. Frequent comments deprecatory to governing agencies can be heard at hospital meetings; they are an exercise in futility. Federal, state, and local controls will only become more pervasive. As government assumes more responsibility for health care reimbursement, the extent and scope of the control will increase.

Christopher W. Bryan-Brown addresses the problem of limited resources and questionable needs in Chapter 2. Too often an ICU is a showplace for the hospital rather than a well-staffed source of progressive and sophisticated care. It is imperative that an institution's needs be honestly assessed and evaluated before proceeding with plans for construction of a specialized unit. A consultant who has no allegiances within the hospital is best equipped to determine if increased critical-care services are needed and, if so, which type is best suited to fulfill that need.

Of the three basic types of intensive/critical-care units, none depends on the physiological problem of the patient population. The first is the intensive nursing unit, which is a modification of the previous method of grouping the sickest patients around the nursing station. The popularity of the intensive nursing unit is based primarily on the highly visible nurse/patient ratio. This type of unit engenders a sense of security for the patient, family, and physician. However, it can be a self-defeating system in that skills, interests, and challenges are removed from the general units, resulting in more beds needed in the intensive nursing unit. Only patients who are potentially or actually physiologically unstable, requiring frequent medical/nursing intervention, should be admitted to ICUs.

General nursing units should have a discrete area for care of the sickest patients in which the nurse/patient ratio is one nurse for two or three patients. This concentrated nursing area will provide experience for the staff in the nursing of the seriously ill patient. Only patients who can benefit from concentrated nursing care and who do not require invasive monitoring should be treated in such areas. Patients transferred from a critical-care unit might be placed in the concentrated nursing area for a transition period before being returned to general floor care.

The second type of unit is the critical-care unit, and the third is the critical-care service. The difference between these two units is primarily one of scope and function. The critical-care service is distinctive for the in-depth involvement of specially trained, full-time physicians and clinical nurse specialists. A critical-care service is most likely to be found in a teaching hospital where patients receive excellent care, and teaching and training for physicians, nurses, and paramedical personnel occur on a regular ongoing basis. Expectations for these units include research programs, innovative approaches to current problems, and a willingness to venture into the unknown. It is to be expected that a critical-care service contributes to the knowledge of critical care by publishing the findings of research and experiences.

The critical-care service provides consultation for seriously ill patients, not only within the institution, but also for critical-care units in the community. The staffs of these critical-care services, as leaders in their field, would be expected to contribute to educational programs and seminars.

The Joint Commission on Accreditation of Hospitals (JCAH) makes no distinction between the critical-care service and the critical-care unit. The critical-care unit adheres to the written regulations of the JCAH, whereas the critical-care service not only meets regulations but surpasses expectations.

When the decision is made concerning the type of unit to be built, the finance division can begin to prepare a budget for operating costs during the first year. Information used in preparing the budget will be obtained from figures available in the geographical area or from the institution itself on the cost of operating a critical-care bed. In subsequent years, the budget can be planned as outlined in Chapter 3 by Stevens.

The furnishings and equipment necessary to begin operating a unit are considered part of the overall cost. Items that cost more than a predetermined, arbitrary amount are part of the capital budget.

Budgeting should reflect the actual projected cost of all personnel, supplies, and equipment for the coming fiscal year as well as a per annum depreciation allotment for capital equipment.

The goal in developing a budget is to accurately itemize costs to have a realistic dollar figure for operating the unit. Many institutions have a tradition of overpricing the budget to cushion against budgetary cuts or as a reserve for unschedualed expenses. This is a waste of time, since the finance department is aware of the practice and simply cuts 10%, or whatever the traditional figure happens to be, from each departmental budget.

Sound fiscal practice dictates that the budget be honestly and accurately constructed. Believable priorities should be designated for equipment purchases. Several authors in this book allude to overequipping the ICU; this is a problem with which we are all familiar. A survey of most units would reveal thousands of dollars worth of machinery standing unused or underused. This is a waste of a limited and valuable resource—money!

Once a budget is approved, the manager has a yardstick by which to measure administrative skills. Few operations are so well-managed that improvement cannot take place. Using equipment and personnel to the fullest advantage is a challenge.

If at the end of the fiscal year the budget has been either overspent or underspent, the manager should scrutinize the entire process, examine the items that did not fall within 5% of the allotment, and determine the reason. If it is the personnel item, census figures may indicate increased or decreased staffing costs. Census figures may also explain a discrepancy in the amount spent for supplies and repairs. Funds remaining in the capital budget may be due to cancellation. With these types of information, appropriate adjustments can be made in subsequent years.

Capital equipment should be assigned a life expectancy at the time of purchase. The expected time of use divided into the cost will give a dollar figure for depreciation each year, and that cost should be included in the annual budget. For instance, if a piece of new equipment cost $10,000 and has a life expectancy of 5 years, $2000 should be allotted annually toward the replacement.

A well-designed budget is a useful tool and should not be looked on as an onerous task to be done in a halfhearted fashion. Actually, only the first year is difficult. All other years, the budget can be built on the previous year with appropriate adjustments.

CHAPTER 1

Feasibility of need

Warren F. Stevens

In the broadest sense, an individual's health is the capacity to maintain a reasonable balance of life activities given one's age and social needs. To maintain this balance, the individual should be free of pain, disease, discomfort, or disabling conditions, thus permitting the enjoyment of a good quality of life and self-fulfillment.

Living habits over time greatly determine an individual's degree of wellness at various ages. Proper rest, relaxation, nutrition, and exercise, when adhered to, can increase longevity. Achieving and maintaining conditions that promote good health are the responsibility of each person.

In everyone's life, situations develop that preclude the actual achievement and maintenance of a state of well-being and health. At this point the individual as a potential patient develops a perceived need for assistance from the health care system. Does the health care system have sufficient service potential to meet the perceived need of the individual? How were these services anticipated and, thus available at the time of the individual need? How was the system able to anticipate the patient's needs and those of others by having the service operational? This chapter examines these questions and explains how to determine the feasibility of need for these services.

HEALTH GOALS

To assist the individual in achieving and maintaining a state of well-being and health, the health system in each community must establish health goals for the inhabitants of that community. Goals and objectives will provide guidance for health care system decision makers in establishing programs and services to meet the community's health needs.

The health goals as written are broad in nature and should be viewed as long-term. Since goals are not usually quantifiable and do not have specific dates for attainment, they provide a general framework for developing the health care system.

An example of typical community health goals necessary for the population to achieve and maintain a state of well-being and health follows:

1. To provide sufficient opportunities for the inhabitants of the area to achieve and maintain the highest possible level of health
2. To provide mechanisms whereby the inhabitants of the area are fully aware of their own rights and responsibilities for achieving and maintaining their own health and the health of others
3. To provide mechanisms whereby the incidence of preventable illness can be reduced
4. To provide mechanisms, where possible, that reduce the mortality and morbidity of unavoidable illness
5. To support activities that reduce environmental health hazards for inhabitants of the area
6. To design, develop, and implement a system of health services, both public and private, that are available, accessible, acceptable, comprehensive, of high quality, efficient, economical, and meet the needs of inhabitants of the area

Thus health goals address the individual's right and responsibility for health maintenance. These goals call for provision of opportunities to permit attainment of health, preventable illness reduction, unavoidable illness reduction, reduction of morbidity and mortality where possible, environmental health concerns, and a system of health services.

OBJECTIVES FOR THE HEALTH CARE DELIVERY SYSTEM

From health goals developed for a community, a series of objectives evolves to support and further delineate the goals. Objectives usually represent targets that the community will work toward over a period of time.

Objectives developed for the health system by a local health system agency (HSA) are as follows[1]:

1. Assure a reasonable distribution of facilities and services to promote accessibility and availability consistent with constraints of reasonable cost, appropriate quality, adequate staffing by competent service providers, and special needs of specific population groups
2. Assure a complete range of services on an around-the-clock basis coordinated by agencies, institutions, and providers
3. Seek to achieve an emergency medical system response time of 5 minutes or less, access to primary and secondary care within 15 to 20 minutes, and access to a tertiary care center within 30 minutes by automobile under normal travel conditions
4. Assure that services provided meet minimum standards of quality as established by local professional standard-setting groups and by the state
5. Assure that services will be efficient and economical for the patient and in terms of the overall economy of the community health system

6. Assure sensitivity to the full range of the patient's needs and rights and those of the family
7. Provide mechanisms for communicating about and resolving problems, complaints, or deficiencies in service
8. Assure the availability of assistance in communicating effectively for persons who speak foreign languages or who have other special communication needs
9. Assure a multilevel system of health services that makes adequately available at the neighborhood or community level a full range of primary services such as ambulatory, preventive and health maintenance, and aftercare services
10. Assure a variety of services and payment mechanisms including both fee for service and prepaid group practices
11. Assure effective patient transportation systems with adequate staffing and proper equipment
12. Assure the development and application of sound planning to the entire system and, more specifically, assure the development of adequate community-wide coordinated planning for:
    a. Emergency medical services
    b. General inpatient acute care
    c. Outpatient care services, both clinical and supportive
    d. Perinatal services
    e. Pediatric services
    f. Critical-care and intensive care services
    g. Long-term care services
    h. Rehabilitation services
    i. Home health services
    j. Cardiac and vascular surgery
    k. Radiation therapy
    l. Renal services
    m. Mental health, alcoholism, and drug abuse services
    n. Services to the developmentally disabled
13. Assure effective use of facilities and services, minimize unnecessary duplication of facilities and services, and promote conversion of underused resources to more appropriate uses
14. Assure adequate financial support and prompt reimbursement for those health resources needed in the community and those which meet the service quality standards established for the community
15. Assure the availability of information services, costs, staff qualifications, and use for each health program
16. Assure the elimination of barriers to service in the health care system, whether the barriers be financial, informational, cultural, social, or conflicts in scheduling
17. Promote incentives for effective service, containing costs, and improving the economy and efficiency of the system

18. Promote appropriate and efficient development and use of manpower and special skills throughout the service system
19. Promote openness to innovations that improve the organization, flexibility, quality, and effectiveness of the system or its component parts
20. Support the implementation of basic and applied research in the health sciences
21. Assure the education of the citizens of the community in matters of health maintenance, preventive care, system use, health care rights and responsibilities, options for care, financing of care, the capabilities and limits of the system and workers in it, and ways to participate in the planning and policy making for the health care system
22. Assure the regular evaluation of services, manpower, administration, and costs, the prompt development of recommendations for resolving problems or removing deficiencies, and the prompt implementation of approved recommendations

These objectives of the health care delivery system constitute what one community views as necessary to maintain and sustain the health of its citizenry.

CONCEPT OF NEED

It is important to differentiate between concepts of need and want. Many times what is initially defined as a need by health care providers actually represents a want of additional equipment and services to deliver a higher quality of care. However, the impact of new services and equipment on the quality of care is subject to question.

Donabedian[2, pp. 62-63] states:

> It is clear that there are at least two perspectives on need: that of the client and that of the provider. . . . The physician's definition of need derives from the manner in which medical science defines health and illness and what medical technology has to offer as treatment or prevention. . . . The client's view of need is likely to differ from that of the physician in a number of ways. . . . First, there is a less complete commitment to the "scientific" view of disease: its causation, evolution and treatment. Residual folk beliefs color the client's view. Second, although the scientific view may be accepted in principle, there is imperfect knowledge of particular diseases as they are scientifically defined. Third, the time horizon of the client tends to be narrower, with emphasis on current manifestations rather than ultimate consequences. . . . Finally, the client is relatively more concerned with the impact of illness in terms of physical discomfort and interference with the activities of successful living as he defines them and as they are defined for him by his place in society. Thus, physician and client are likely to define health in terms of different dimensions.

The concept of need then is "applied to (a) states of health or ill health, (b) use of service, and (c) levels of supply."[2, p. 65]

ASSESSMENT OF NEED PROCESS

To assess the need of a proposed service or support equipment, it is necessary to examine the basis behind the assessment process itself. It is anticipated that the health care system will make a difference in patient outcomes. Thus, the assessment process should be able to define that a positive differentiation in health status will occur as a result of a specific treatment. When various courses of treatment are available for a specific disease, the treatment that provides the greatest positive differentiation in health status should receive priority. When all diseases and their respective selected treatments are considered collectively on a community-wide basis, treatments that have the most impact on patient outcome and health status should receive the highest priority.

To determine priorities as specified, it is essential that a series of health status indicators be used. An information basis for this determination will include the population by age-specific categories; the morbidity of the population; the mortality of the population; situations requiring health care system intervention not previously defined; and the general health status of the population.

An assessment of need process can be used in many ways. It provides feedback on the health care system, which indicates partial success or failure of the system interface with patients. In addition to the system interface, many influences have an impact on and account for the overall condition of patients.

The assessment of need process can also be used to establish priorities. Assessment, then, is an essential condition to the planning process. In the planning process, once priorities have been set, objectives for health care service needs can be determined.

When the objectives are set, they can be further specified into units of service. The service units are then translated into resources necessary to satisfy health needs from the assessment process. The assessment of need process constitutes the basis of decision making for new services for the health care system.

Measures of health and illness

To perform an assessment of need properly, it is essential that measures of health and illness be developed for this process. In planning health care services, the information most commonly used is the population size and its demographic characteristics. These measures will normally include socioeconomic factors and geographical attributes. This information can be secured from the periodic census taken by the federal government.

Another common measure of health and illness is mortality. Most communities have complete records on mortality. With increased awareness of chronic diseases, the use of mortality as the principal indicator of health has diminished. Since this phenomenon has occurred, emphasis has been placed more on measures of morbidity and disability. Certainly, obtaining information about sickness levels and restriction of activity aids the patient and health care system in general by approaching problems earlier in the disease process.

Other measures of health and illness are not readily apparent from mortality or morbidity indicators. Basically, they are situations that require health care but cannot be considered as morbidity or mortality indicators. This aspect of need represents the prevention of illness and maintenance of health. These need levels include routine physical examinations as well as delivery care services such as well baby and child care clinics.

California Community Health Systems Analysis and Evaluation Model

In 1972 the California State Office of Comprehensive Health Planning developed and issued a document entitled "California Community Health Systems Analysis and Evaluation Model." This model was designed to address "methodology and data sets to be employed in estimating the resource requirements for the effective, efficient, and equitable delivery of health services to community populations."[3, p.1]

Briefly, the model estimates resource requirements based on service needs of the population studied. The report provided the following description of methodology.[3, pp. 5-6]

Step 1. *Determine population* of geographic area under consideration. (The population should be broken down by various demographic and socioeconomic variables.)

Step 2. *Estimate morbidity in population.* In order to be able to link conditions in the population to service requirements, morbidity must be described by the International Standard Classification of Disease since it is currently the only available index which is used to describe both definite and differential diagnoses. The morbidity rates should be based on various demographic and socioeconomic variables (age, sex, race, etc).

Step 3. *Estimate service needs.* This requires delineation of the types of health services and settings and an estimate of volume of services by type and setting. For example, in the case of physicians, services would be described as office visits, home visits, consultations, etc. Estimates of volume of services would be made for each type of service by diagnostic category.

Step 4. *Participation rates by occupation.* For each type of service, estimates need to be made of the percentage of services performed by the relevant health occupations. For example, calculations have to be made for all maternity services with respect to the percentage performed by general practitioners and by obstetricians.

Step 5. *Productivity rates.* For each health occupation, productivity rates have to be calculated.

Step 6. *Calculation of manpower needs.* This is done by dividing productivity rates into the estimated number of services delivered by the respective health occupations.

Step 7. *Calculation of facility needs.* This is done by extracting the inpatient portion of the total service needs (expressed in terms of number of inpatient days per diagnostic category and type of admission) and dividing the days in the year adjusted by a standard occupancy differential.

Step 8. *Comparison with health service capacity.* After the various estimates and projections of service requirements have been made, the last step is a comparison of the capacity of the health system to deliver the necessary services.

This model is one example of methodologies that can be used by health planning agencies to assess needs in a community and to determine what services are required to meet those needs.

Levels of health service specialization

In each community, health services tend to be grouped according to levels of complexity or specialization. Grouping by levels of specialization facilitates the understanding and analysis of health services. This approach permits health care programs to be organized according to the intensity of service to be delivered to the patient. Thus, each community examines its services based on the following three levels of specialization:

Primary care—This level, which is usually entry level for the patient, provides services of a noncritical nature. Primary care can include routine outpatient care, preventive care, diagnosis and treatment, rehabilitation services, and patient education service.

Secondary care—This level of care is intermediate in specialization. Secondary care usually is provided in general community hospitals as standard inpatient care. Patients for this level of care are referred by office-based, specialized physicians.

Tertiary care—This level of care is the most specialized available to patients; it occurs in regional medical centers and specialty hospitals. Tertiary care is expensive, requires highly educated proficient practitioners, and uses complicated treatment procedures.

This discussion will be limited to tertiary care, and in some cases, secondary care. Critical-care services meet conditions of tertiary care, but in practice are often delivered at general community hospitals. The following case illustrates critical-care feasibility of need. The area of concern will be the feasibility of need for open heart surgery services.

CRITICAL-CARE FEASIBILITY OF NEED—OPEN HEART SURGERY

Within the concept of levels of specialization, open heart surgery is a tertiary care service. As previously mentioned, tertiary care should occur at a regional medical center or specialty hospital. Open heart surgery is a complicated treatment procedure involving highly specialized manpower and extensive equipment; it is a high-cost service.

Initially, a planning agency will collect information about the current incidence of cardiac surgery in the community or county. This information reveals the number of medical centers performing open heart surgery and the number of cases at each institution over a period of time. Data of this nature include the following:

- Ten of forty hospitals in area perform open heart surgery
- 800 open heart surgeries were performed during the calendar year 1976
- An increase of 100 surgeries was noted over the calendar year 1975
- On the average, ten hospitals averaged eighty surgeries an institution during the calendar year 1976
- Current minimum number of cases each year should be 150[4]

In addition, information regarding the number of physicians practicing under specialties of thoracic surgery and cardiovascular surgery is obtained from local physician directories. These figures provide initial estimates of physician manpower available to the area. Data of this nature include the following:

- Forty physicians practice thoracic surgery
- Twenty physicians practice cardiovascular surgery
- Eighteen physicians practicing thoracic surgery are also listed under cardiovascular surgery

Next, trends in the specialty are examined. The planning agency examines standards for that service, if standards are available on a local and national basis. In the case of open heart surgery, professional standards such as the following are available:

Hospital Categorization Guidelines: Optimal Criteria for Hospital Resources for the Care of Patients with Heart Disease, Cancer, Stroke, and End-Stage Kidney Disease, Joint Commission on Accreditation of Hospitals, 1974.

Cardiovascular Diseases, Guidelines for Prevention and Care, the Inter-Society Commission for Heart Disease Resources, 1972.

These standards will be interpreted on a community level with guidelines for local decision makers. To ensure quality patient care, guidelines for staffing and equipment for open heart surgery may be written:

Open heart surgical team
- Board-certified or board-eligible thoracic surgeon with specialized education and experience in open heart surgery will have overall responsibility for open heart surgical team. (Sometimes experience is specified in terms of the number of surgeries, such as 150 or 200.)
- Two additional surgeons (one board-certified or board-eligible) will be required as a minimum.
- Board-certified or board-eligible cardiologist will assist as a surgical team member in monitoring the patient.
- Board-certified or board-eligible anesthesiologist will administer anesthesia to open heart surgery patients.
- Clinical perfusionists will operate extracorporeal equipment under supervision of a surgeon or cardiologist.

Nursing staff
- One or two scrub nurses and one or two circulating nurses with special education and experience in cardiac surgery will assist during open heart surgery.

- Qualified critical-care nurses will provide nursing care to patients in the postoperative cardiac care unit. Staffing will permit one nurse for one patient during each shift.

Allied health personnel
- Sufficient allied health personnel with appropriate credentials, education, and experience will be present on each shift to support treatment procedures required by open heart surgery patients.

Equipment
- Equipment will meet standards developed by the state.
- Surgical suites will be established to permit the dedication of at least one suite for open heart surgery.
- Cardiac catheterization laboratory will be an integral part of open heart surgery care. The laboratory will be located where the surgery is performed. To maintain proper quality of care, at least 250 to 300 procedures should be performed each year.
- Blood bank and pulmonary function laboratory should be available on a 24-hour basis. Blood gas determination and pH determination capabilities should be immediately available to both surgical suites and catheterization laboratory.
- Postoperative cardiac care unit, equipped as an ICU/CCU, should be available and separated from the coronary care unit and general ICU.
- Emergency medical service transportation should be available on a 24-hour basis with the capability to stabilize patients before and during transport.
- Numerous support services, such as electrocardiography, vectorcardiography, echocardiography, phonocardiography, cardiac rehabilitation, and pulse tracing are usually suggested.

Once the data have been collected and standards have been established in terms of guidelines, population projections are made by age-specific categories. Each age category has an experienced incidence of coronary problems. From the number of individuals projected for each category, a coronary incidence projection can be made, and community aggregate can be determined to establish a need level for 1985, for example. These projections are based on the assumption that life-styles will not change substantially and that advances in medical technology have been taken into consideration, given current knowledge.

Thus, the projected incidence and standards for quality patient care are examined to secure a system that can deliver effective and efficient care. A calculation of need would be:

$$\frac{\text{Projected patient case load}}{\substack{\text{Minimum number of cases} \\ \text{to deliver quality patient care}}} = \substack{\text{Maximum number of medical} \\ \text{centers that should have units}}$$

$$\frac{1050 \text{ cases}}{150 \text{ cases}} = \text{Seven medical centers}$$

Therefore, based on current projections to 1985, only seven medical centers should be offering open heart surgery in our hypothetical community. Since the 150-case load is on a team basis, this aspect must be examined in a final determination. In this situation, if ten hospitals are offering open heart surgery, the system has excess service capacity, and no need for additional units exists. It would be strongly recommended that some of the existing open heart surgery services be consolidated to not exceed the community need for open heart surgery. The same type of approach could be used wherever the minimum number of cases required to maintain team proficiency has been determined.

CONCLUSION

It must be remembered in determining need that the mere offering of services does not represent a need for those services. Both health care providers and consumers have a responsibility to provide community-identified health care in a cost-effective manner.

REFERENCES

1. Report A-1 of the Orange County health services plan: framework for an area health system, Tustin, Calif., 1975, Orange County Health Planning Council, pp. 26-28.
2. Donabedian, A.: Aspects of medical care administration: specifying requirements for health care, Cambridge, Mass., 1973, Harvard University Press.
3. California community health systems analysis and evaluation model, San Francisco, 1972, California State Office of Comprehensive Health Planning, Program Analysis and Evaluation Bureau.
4. California Administrative Code, Title 22, Division 5, Section 20433.

BIBLIOGRAPHY

Alexander, T.: Multihospital system may offer solutions to delivery problems, Hospitals **50**(21):73-76, 1976.

California community health systems analysis and evaluation model, San Francisco, 1972, California State Office of Comprehensive Health Planning, Program Analysis and Evaluation Bureau.

Cardiovascular diseases: Guidelines for prevention and care, New York, 1972, Inter-Society Commission for Heart Disease Resources.

Donabedian, A.: Aspects of medical care administration: specifying requirements for health care, Cambridge, Mass., 1973, Harvard University Press.

Harmon, G. J.: Start planning by defining the community, its future needs, Hospitals **50**(12):105-109, 112, 1976.

Holloway, R. G.: Planning for results and specific outcomes, Hospitals **50**(10):77-82, 1976.

Hospital categorization guidelines: optimal criteria for hospital resources for the care of patients with heart disease, cancer, stroke, and end-stage kidney disease, Chicago, 1974, Joint Commission on Accreditation of Hospitals.

Phillips, D. F.: Research aims at influencing health care policy and delivery, Hospitals **51**(7):55-60, 1977.

Report A-1 of the Orange County health services plan: framework for an area health system, Tustin, Calif, 1975, Orange County Health Planning Council, pp. 26-28.

Schultz, R., and Johnson, A. C.: Management of hospitals, New York, 1976, McGraw-Hill Book Co.

CHAPTER 2

Project management

Christopher W. Bryan-Brown

The cost of critical care is adding substantially to escalating costs of hospital medicine. The large amount of medical resources required for the setting up and running of ICUs in a fully effective manner is beyond the financial capabilities of many institutions. It is possible for one fourth of the budget of a hospital nursing department to be expended on the treatment of less than 5% of the patients. Without intensive care some would die, but many do in spite of it. A unit improperly set up and managed is a frequent occurrence in hospitals that feel obliged to run one for the sake of completeness or prestige, but do not have the priority to staff or equip it adequately. The result is often increased cost with slight patient benefit. High mortality rates in ICUs can make them appear to squander on hopeless enterprise. Insurance companies and government agencies do not find great appeal in expending large sums of money for inadequate or inappropriate care.

The ICU may be the birthplace of treatments that can be later applied to patients outside, but already technological advances have outstripped the community's willingness to pay for them. Medicine commands over 8% of the gross national product, which has prompted many community spokesmen from political and consumer groups to question the fiscal responsibility of those within the medical profession. The delivery of health care appears inefficient and lacking self-discipline when increased costs go unchecked. Legislation to contain these costs, while maintaining high medical standards, has been enacted. Regulations from local, state, and federal health departments now guide and coerce those who deliver health care. The effect of some of these regulations on the setting up and running of ICUs is discussed in this chapter.

PLANNING LEGISLATION

The National Health Planning and Resources Development Act of 1974 (PL 93-641) governs much of the regulatory process to evaluate the need for

15

increased institutional services and permit their development when a substantial increase in medical costs is anticipated as a result. (Nonsubstantial projects are often considered to be those of less than $100,000 a year, but no actual sum has been legally defined.) The act called on local areas with a population of 500,000 to 3,000,000 to formulate health systems plans (HSPs) and associated annual implementation plans. The states are expected to cooperate with the local HSPs to produce an overall State Health Plan (SHP) to be run by the Statewide Health Coordinating Council (SHCC) and controlled by the state health planning and development agency. The demands of authorities vary from basic adherence to the act to tougher, long-term requirements. The latter tend to be in areas in which many tertiary facilities are centered. In Massachusetts, all hospitals submit both one- and five-year plans for capital expenditure, and permission to develop a new program (certificate of need) cannot be requested for items not in the plan for that year.

The Council (SHCC) has a legally specified composition and responsibility. The governor appoints 60% of its members from the state's health systems agencies; they have a consumer majority. The inclusion of consumerists may not be helpful. This element in the development of new projects may give rise to protracted negotiation. To quote Lasagna[1]:

> How these persons are chosen and whom they represent is not clear. But it is evident that some highly influential consumerist advocates speak for themselves rather than as a result of a specific mandate from a large constituency. These persons are often passionate, dedicated, skillful expositors, as well as masters of dramatic overstatement.

A task of the Council is to review HSPs and annual implementation plans. The state agency administers the approval process for new programs and reviews new institutional health services. It is duty bound to make public its findings. Because other state agencies may perform any of the ascribed functions at the request of the governor (under an agreement with the state agency and to the satisfaction of the Secretary of Health, Education, and Welfare), considerable variations in the approach have developed from state to state.

In addition, the Health Systems Agencies (HSA) become involved when federal funding is requested. These operate both at state and local levels. When applications for new programs are made to the state agency, they are passed on to both the local and state planning agencies and the HSA. Public notice is made for the proposed program so that interested parties can make known their views. If the application is turned down, a public hearing may be held, and evidence concerning the need for services can be aired openly. In the event of a favorable decision, a certificate of need is then granted to the applying institution. The program may be implemented provided that budgetary limits are not exceeded. Compliance with these regulatory agencies is greatly enhanced by their control of reimbursement.

DEVELOPING AN ICU

The stages of developing an ICU should follow a process of project management (Fig. 2-1). Each stage in the scheme must be documented, and decisions made before proceeding to the next. It cannot be emphasized too often that great efforts have to be made to convince various public bodies and key private individuals that an intensive care unit is needed. When the public relations side of the plan is well-handled there is often less difficulty in wading through the bureaucratic maze that stands between perception of a need and proof of that need. The collection and presentation of verifiable data by substantial people go a long way in effecting the progress of a plan when it reaches the public sector.

Formation

The possibility that an ICU might be beneficial is expressed as an initiating request. At this point, there is no commitment of either personnel or money. Much of the early stage is done informally, often by a small group of protagonists who try to persuade the hospital administration to make an institutional commitment to the project.

At this early stage some data are needed to show how the ICU will improve patient care. This frequently takes the form of a catalogue of disasters

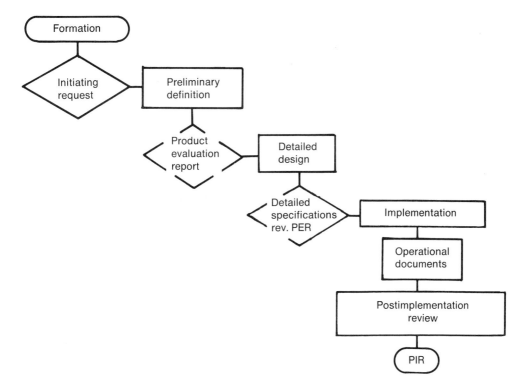

Fig. 2-1. Project management process.

that might have been avoided if special care facilities had been available. A short survey of the mortality rate of patients receiving ventilation therapy, proportion of patients who die after a craniotomy, or an increase in the activity of an accident service in an emergency department are the sort of figures that help justification. A cold account of the cases that involve the hospital in large damage suits for medical liability that might have been avoided if the proposed unit had been in existence often has much emotional as well as fiscal impact.

A search should be made for potential support both from within and outside the hospital. The logistical key to patient management in an ICU is critical-care nursing. Involvement of the nursing department at this stage is not only sound medically, but is good political ammunition later because it will be looked for by the various government agencies that are needed to give approval for the project. Token input from the nursing department is usually resented by that department and is quick to be spotted by an examining authority. Support from various other departments should be solicited with a view to future aid. Some of these are biomedical engineering, laboratory services, respiratory therapy, and various involved chiefs of medical departments for the provision of medical coverage. Outside the hospital interest of various sympathetic community groups should be solicited. A quest for charitable sources of funding at this point may also indicate where political support lies. It is often much easier to convince an institution that a new facility is worthwhile if a governmental or philanthropic source of funding can be found. If this campaign is successful, then a preliminary definition is made.

Preliminary definition

This is the phase when the feasibility of developing the ICU is worked out. It ends with a product evaluation report. The director of the hospital or relevant department should now set up an ICU planning committee. This should preferably be chaired by someone who has both established experience in critical care and medical politics. Members of the committee should be able to make decisions on behalf of their departments, since frequent references to other authority is time consuming. The designated medical director and representatives from the departments of nursing, hospital planning, and finance should be included. A good first step is to visit other institutions with ICUs that serve the same purpose as the proposed one. This visit can then be followed by visits from acknowledged experts in critical care who review the institution's requirements and make suggestions how they might best be met. Since medical, nursing, and hospital planning expertise of sufficient caliber is not frequently found together in one institution, outside help will usually save many planning errors later. Space allocation and the impact of losing or gaining beds have to be among initial considerations.

Early contact should be made with the planning authorities, SHCC and HSA, informing them that application for a certificate of need is being considered and soliciting their advice. It is politically wise to have a clinician, such as a chief of service or a designated ICU medical director, available from the beginning to speak to local interest groups. The public relations aspect of a physician involved in the critical-care needs of the community can counter some of the antiorganized medicine faction among the consumer advocates. Support from local politicians and citizens' organizations is helpful for convincing health planning agencies of the need for a new program. This early-warning and informal politicking has become an integral component of the negotiating system.

Another factor in the negotiating process is the institutional record of compliance to the requests of health planning agencies. A hospital with a good reputation has already established credibility. Other requirements of health planning may also be part of the bargaining. For instance, a hospital planning goal is to reduce the number of acute beds in a community to four for each thousand of population. Agencies may start the negotiations, in the case of a larger institution, with the question of reduction of maximum patient census if a new substantial project is to be allowed.

Although the goal for health agencies in reducing the hospital beds of the community to an economically more acceptable number has been set, that for critical-care facilities has not. Institutional needs have to be justified by data. The number and use of existing ICU beds, the number of patients not admitted to an ICU, but requiring critical care, and the hospital plan for care of critically ill patients in the absence of ICU beds will all be needed as evidence. The justification of small ICUs is difficult, and an overall examination of the institution may suggest that a grouping of facilities by various medical services would best meet the needs and be more economical. Unless an institution is small and no other facilities are available in the area, it is unlikely that a health agency would normally approve an application for an ICU of much less than eight beds. If an institution can show a need for about twice this number then a stand alone ICU becomes more economically justifiable.

Feasibility studies have to be produced to predict the financial impact on the institution, third-party reimbursement, and the availability of adequate funds. Space allocation and compliance to hospital codes and agency standards require help from planners and architects. The technical aspects, projected staffing patterns with suitable training programs and direction, have to be assessed both with a view to fiscal and personnel resource availability.

When the data and broad plans are ready, and supportive community groups have been appraised of the application, legal and jurisdictional feasibility is then sought by obtaining the permission (certificate of need) to proceed from the various external agencies, such as health departments, HSA, and SHCC. When a permission is obtained, a product evaluation report is generated, and the decision to continue into a phase of detailed design can be made.

Detailed design

This phase is the development of detailed plans for the project. Failure to make a sufficiently detailed and comprehensive design usually leads to unnecessary alterations and expense later. It is here that the expertise of the planning committee comes to the fore. Final architectural plans are made, bids put out to tender, and requests for equipment bids are solicited and reviewed.

Appropriate evaluation of apparatus is made, preferably within the institution, but if this is not possible, the evaluation is based on samples in action elsewhere. Final decisions on most apparatus selection will depend on servicing and availability. A contract should include specifications such as installation and conditions under which the buyer will consider the apparatus acceptable. Detailed plans will be needed for the staffing and supply of backup facilities and for material for day-to-day patient management within the unit. It is usually very expensive to make changes in management of the project after this point. Therefore it is incumbent on the planning committee to predict and meet the requirements of potential users of the ICU in as much detail as possible.

There is also an appropriate point to solicit the generosity of a philanthropist who may wish to be memorialized by having his or her name bestowed on an impressive hospital facility. This line of additional support is not available for government agency–operated institutions. Unfortunately, these latter tend to work with planning departments without enough skill or competence to provide an appropriate unit.

One of the dangers in any ICU planning is overkill. Massive computerization and monitoring are seldom used to capacity and are very expensive. When the American Hospital Asociation (AHA) surveyed special care facilities, it was found that only a fraction of patients in these units required full, critical-care support. In general for ICUs of the fourteen- to twenty-bed range, it is unlikely that more than about one third of the beds should be fully monitored for multisystem failure patients. Other facilities such as the acute areas of accident units receiving patients with multiple trauma have a much higher need. Without taking this type of consideration into account, much money can be wasted on equipment that will never be used. It is important to have areas that can be scaled down during the implementation phase to keep the budget within predictive cost. Completion is documented by detailed specifications. The product evaluation report will have to be reviewed to ensure that detailed specifications cover the full scope of the project and keep within budgetary limits. If cost increases are considered nonsubstantial by the health planning agencies, the project may then be implemented.

Implementation

Constructing and equipping the ICU, staffing, and the development of protocols and standards according to the detailed specifications are then implemented. This is the time when policies for unit management have to be written and passed by the various departments concerned and the medical board of the hospital. The medical demands are that the duties of the medical director and the named deputy be spelled out. The relationship and responsibilities of unit medical staff and physicians referring patients to the ICU must be defined. Policies for admission and discharge must be decided on in conjunction with other units in the hospital to make sure that critical care is available to all patients who might need it. Policies and procedures have to be developed to define what procedures may be done in the unit and who may do them. Plans should be made for education and training of staff.

The unit medical director should appoint an ICU committee. This should include the supervisor or head nurse of the unit, representation from any department that may make any major call on the services of the unit, and such persons as biomedical engineers and respiratory therapists who may be involved in the day-to-day running of the unit. One of the charges of this committee is to write and maintain up-to-date policies, procedures, and standards for the operation of the unit. It should be responsible either to relevant department chiefs or the medical board of the hospital. Another useful function of this committee is the development of budget priorities. Once the unit is set up, this committee should have a full meeting at least every 3 months.

During the phase of implementation the planning committee has to show considerable self-discipline because the temptation to change things becomes great. It is here that the value of the committee's work in the phase of detail design becomes apparent. Alterations at this point should be kept to a minimum, but practice is different, especially by those who do not understand project management. A problem in critical care is that patient management and equipment change so fast, few ICUs can be constructed before some of the detailed specifications have become outdated. This phase is complete when operational documents are produced.

Postimplementation review

The project should be reviewed after completion to ascertain whether original goals were met, and to ascertain if and why differences arose. Postimplementation review is good project management practice and may become a requirement of health planning agencies when substantial increases in costs are incurred.

REFERENCE

1. Lasagna, L.: Wanted: new type of consumer advocate for drugs, N. Engl. J. Med. **298:**906, 1978.

CHAPTER 3

The budget

Warren F. Stevens

Every professional in critical care is interested in quality patient care. The quality of patient care depends on the effective use of human and nonhuman resources. When health care costs are limited or restricted, the availability of resources is curtailed. In this type of situation, which is typical today, the stress to improve the effective use of resources is not a choice but a necessity.

A common misconception in critical care and health care in general is that the day-to-day costs of running a critical-care unit or hospital are totally controlled by hospital administration and department heads. The fact is that each employee on every level of the organization has responsibility for the greatest part of the operational budget. Working each day in a critical-care unit, employees use supplies and resources to deliver patient care. Through this process, the time spent working in the unit is translated into patient costs in terms of payroll and benefits for employees as well as the cost of supplies and other resources consumed for patient care. These items collectively account for the greatest amount of hospital and critical-care budgets and costs.

OPERATIONAL BUDGETS
General considerations

The nurse manager in the critical-care unit plans, organizes, directs, and controls activities that account for the vast majority of expenses incurred by the unit. Where does the money come from to pay salary, supply, and equipment costs? The funds come from patient bills for services rendered through the hospital organization. Those bills are paid by the patient directly or through third-party payors, such as insurance companies, Blue Cross, Medicaid, and Medicare funds. In most cases, the physician is the activating source for bringing the patient to the hospital with the exception of some emergencies. Through the identification of an illness requiring treatment, the physician admits the patient. From that point, the hospital accrues income through its billing process to pay for care services delivered to the patient. Thus, the physician is the principal revenue-producing source for the institution. For this reason, from a financial point of view, maintaining the viability of a hospital requires a large active medical staff to ensure a continuous flow of funds to keep services in place to meet patient needs.

How do the hospital administrator, director of nursing, and nurse manager know how much money will be available to pay salaries and purchase supplies? The truth is that they do not know exactly; however, reasonable estimates can be made to anticipate what will happen over the next year. The estimates constitute the budget, a plan for the future. The budget establishes allocation of resources based on projected activities.

Individuals who are exposed to budgets for the first time usually experience a certain amount of cerebral trauma. The following questions are common to this situation: How can I determine how many patients we will have next year? How many patients will need coronary care? How can I predict what will happen? The fact is that fairly accurate estimates can be made.

Even though a budget is a plan for the future, much can be learned by reviewing patient census by disease over the past few years. This information gives an average over time, and indicates trends that can be extrapolated for future planning. Of course, this kind of projection implies that many of the conditions will remain the same. In an overall sense, more factors tend to remain the same than change.

"Although budgets are usually associated with financial statements, such as revenue and expenses, there may be nonfinancial statements covering outputs, materials, and equipment."[1] Usually the specific time for budgets is the fiscal year. Most hospitals use a fiscal year that starts July 1 and ends June 30 of each year. The nonfinancial aspects of budgeting include identifying the level of personnel needed in terms of education and experience, number of personnel in each category, work hours, nurse-patient interaction hours, kinds and amounts of supplies and material to be used, expected hours of equipment use, and the amount of space to be used. The determination of these nonfinancial factors is based on past experience, trends, and available knowledge about the future that may affect the operations of the unit. Variables that may influence future budgeting are the addition of physicians to the medical staff that would increase the census of the unit; a hospital closing in the area, which could divert patients to your hospital for care; or a new surgical procedure that may reduce the length of patient stay by 40%. Therefore, the more information that can be collected, the greater the accuracy of the estimates.

Nonfinancial considerations should be developed prior to the development of financial budgets. Once nonfinancial aspects of budgets have been determined, financial budgets can be priced out. This means that each activity item will be assigned a cost. Each level of personnel will be given salary and employee benefit costs for the year. Consideration of the following aspects is essential to securing an accurate estimate for budgetary purposes: staffing pattern to be used, nursing hours for each patient a day (including professional and nonprofessional nursing hours), calculations based on the hospital work-week, absenteeism, holiday time, staff development, sick time, and vacations. Materials and supplies are assigned costs based on volume of use expected as well as prices provided by vendors. It is important to realize that the number of personnel, level of personnel, and employee benefits are controllable costs, as are materials and supplies. The term controllable costs means that the nurse manager, through the decision-making process, has a certain degree of control over the costs in these areas.

In contrast, noncontrollable costs are costs over which the nurse manager has little, if any control. These costs are usually for overhead items such as utilities (heating, cooling, lighting, gas), allocated portion of mortgage payments, and depreciation on equipment. In many cases, the allocated portion of mortgage payments is based on the amount of floor space that the unit contains in relation to the total square footage of other areas in the hospital.

Thus, in the budgetary process, activity levels as well as costs must be projected as part of the plan. In the operational environment other considerations are necessary to maintain the relevancy of operational budgets. These special considerations will now be examined.

Special considerations

The approach used to determine operational budgets works well in general providing that hospitals receive a relatively consistent flow of funds throughout the year. However, this situation does not always occur as planned. A recently reported situation demonstrates this point. "Anxious nursing home and hospital administrators called Thursday for quick resolution of a Medicaid contract dispute that is tying up more than $3.3 million they are due for treating low-income patients. . . . Switchboards at the state office were swamped Thursday with calls from concerned hospitals and other health care providers—some complaining that they urgently needed their checks in order to meet their payrolls."[2]

Cash budgets. Since the flow of funds is not always consistent, it is commonly suggested that hospitals develop what are known as *cash budgets*. These budgets specifically address the expected flow of funds. The timing of the receipt of funds is most important. It is essential that the flow of funds coming into the hospital coincide with funds being expended for payroll, employee benefits, supplies, and materials. Therefore, in the budgeting process it is necessary to consider and anticipate seasonal fluctuations. Appropriate anticipation of these variations will provide sufficient funds to remain in a liquid position and will demonstrate that the nurse manager is effective in budgeting. Most of the excess funds that occur from time to time using this approach can be invested and earn interest until they are needed to meet expenses.

Flexible budgets. Many nurse managers have become somewhat more sophisticated in their budgeting processes. They realize that some costs are controllable and others are noncontrollable. It is apparent that certain costs are fixed, which means they will not change regardless of unit activity and patient census. On the other hand, they also know that some costs will change depending on patient load and related activity. For these reasons some nurse managers have used what are known as *flexible budgets.* With this type of budgeting, the nurse manager will develop a budget as previously indicated. This budget will be the one most likely to occur. For example, based on average of past activity, census, trends, and future information the budget may be predicated on a 70% occupancy level. To be able to anticipate alternatives that may occur in the future, the nurse manager may also prepare budgets for a 65% level, a 75% level, and an 80% level. In all of these budgets the fixed costs will remain the same. However, at the 65% level, the amount of variable costs will be lower because activity levels will be lower. In a similar fashion, the 75% and the 80% levels will show progressively increased variable costs above the 70% level. If one of these alternative situations begins to develop, the nurse manager already has a budget plan of action to be able to anticipate the changing costs with the changes in the activity level.

For the budgets to be meaningful, expenditures and revenue should be monitored for variations on a periodic basis. Most hospitals have a monthly budgetary review in which all variations need to be explained in writing. Many times the variations indicate cost areas that need additional attention and control. These can be the basis for administrative action to correct situations and bring costs into line with budget projections. In other cases variations that actually represent changes in activity and delivery may reasonably justify a revision in the budget to incorporate these changes adequately.

Moving budgets. Many nurse managers find that attempting to forecast future events is most difficult because of the rapidly changing variables in their work environments. In these types of situations nurse managers have found that moving budgets have been most helpful. In the moving budget concept, the length of time may still be 1 year, but the budget is adjusted at the conclusion of each month by dropping the last month from the budget and adding a new month 1 year ahead. This process represents an annual budget that is revised on a monthly basis. The approach suggested here is time consuming and costly to prepare, but may be an appropriate approach if the variations in the environment are of sufficient magnitude to justify its use.

CAPITAL EXPENDITURE BUDGETS

Previously we have examined the concept of operational budgets. These budgets do not provide for the purchase of major items of equipment or for the addition of physical facilities. For purposes of discussion we will only consider equipment items.

Each year all departments in the hospital submit requests for puchases of equipment to replace old, outmoded equipment or to obtain newly introduced equipment that can enhance the quality of care delivered to patients. In most cases, the equipment identified is expected to be used for the next 5 to 10 years, and for this reason the planning cycle for this type of budget is significantly longer than for 1-year operational budgets.

In preparing capital expenditure budgets for the unit, the nurse manager prepares materials to justify the requests. Managers include information on each item noting manufacturer, model, purchase, delivery, installment and maintenance costs and any special considerations that may be needed. Rating scales are used, and priorities are assigned before submitting the budget to the administration. Rating scales include such levels as urgent, essential, necessary, and helpful. Priorities are then assigned within these rating scales where possible. Usually the administration performs an overall rating of requests for all departments and through action of the board of trustees approves all priority items within available funds for purchases of equipment. Many nurse managers become frustrated with these decisions when only items determined to be urgent are approved for purchase. However, it must be remembered that limited funds are available, the decisions are difficult, and the availability of funds appears to be even more limited in the future.

BUDGETARY PROCESS

Thus far, we have discussed operational budgets, both general and special considerations, as well as capital expenditure budgets. Now we shall examine the budgetary process that culminates in the finalization of operational budgets.

The development of annual operational plans for hospitals usually takes about 1 year prior to the implementation of the plan itself. Most hospitals will have a long-range plan of 3 to 5 years. Each year an annual plan is developed for operations. This plan is to be our concern.

First, long-range goals of the hospital are reviewed and from these long-range goals, short-term objectives are determined for the fiscal year under consideration. General goals of the department of nursing are translated into objectives for the department and its various units, including critical care. These objectives constitute part of the overall management-by-objectives program used by many hospitals in the United States.

Second, each unit and the hospital in general conduct an appraisal of organizational performance. This review includes comparison of past performance with objectives established for those areas. Targets that have been met or exceeded are examined. Likewise, areas of deficiency are reviewed. From these processes strengths and weaknesses are defined, and limitations and other factors that could impede attainment of objectives are identified. At this step in the budgetary process internal use of resources is reviewed, and external factors that might have an impact on operations are considered. This information collectively permits the statement of premises from which future planning will be based. For example, an external factor could be the opening of a new hospital with a full range of services that could reduce overall patient census.

Once these aspects of planning are completed, the individual units, through their nurse managers, can work to define unit objectives. These specific objectives are measurable and quantitative in nature. Through the approval of capital expenditure budgets, these objectives will state the equipment to be purchased for each month, when it will be installed, and when it will be operational. In addition, objectives will include staffing changes anticipated, staff development programs to be offered, preparations for JCAH accreditation visits, development of critical-care nursing standards for the unit, and implementation of an increase in bed capacity for the critical-care unit.

With the development of objectives for the critical-care units, it is essential to delineate the strategies that will be used to implement the objectives and make them a reality. For example, the unit may want to increase overall patient census by 10% during the next year. The following strategies increase efforts to attract more patients to the hospital: working more closely with staff physicians to upgrade patient teaching programs, coordinating plans with hospital admissions to expedite patient flow, and developing greater community awareness of the unit through a public relations program.

At this point the administration makes projections of revenue, and each department develops its activity plan for operations for the year. This nonfinancial portion of the process for units includes staffing levels, nurse/patient interaction hours, kinds and amounts of supplies and materials, hours equipment is expected to be used, and the amount of space to be used.

Next, the activities are costed for each item for each unit. Time of staff is costed by current and projected salary levels, and appropriate employee benefits are assigned. Likewise, materials and supplies are costed as well as equipment and space determinations. The budget is prepared to permit the unit to meet the objectives established for the year. At this point the budgets of all units are submitted for review and revision by the administration. After administrative review, the budgets are submitted to the board of trustees for review and approval. The culmination of a year-long process has resulted in the approval of an operational plan and a budget for the hospital, its departments, and units.

NURSE MANAGER'S FINANCIAL RESPONSIBILITY

The importance of the nurse manager's financial responsibility cannot be overemphasized. Some examples of the magnitude of this level of responsibility will greatly clarify this point. Following is an example of typical financial information compiled from various medical centers:

Fiscal year 1978

Total medical center budget	$30,000,000
Total nursing department budget	$12,000,000

The departments of nursing budgets usually account for 40% to 50% of the total operational budget. Critical-care units are likewise responsible for a significant amount of budgetary expenditures. Actual budget amounts for critical-care units in one medical center for fiscal year 1978 (Fig. 3-1) are given:

Unit	Amount
Neonatal intensive care unit	$ 138,708
E-5	296,279
Coronary care unit	288,873
E-4	296,289
D-4	172,982
Intensive care unit	712,393
Cardiovascular unit	138,115
Emergency room	830,487
Recovery room	398,307
TOTAL CRITICAL-CARE BUDGET	$3,272,433

Thus it is obvious that the nursing director of critical-care units has a significant financial responsibility. Similarly, each unit director is responsible for a budget exceeding $138,000.

CONCLUSION

Health care in the United States has grown as a service industry. It is now considered by many experts to be the first or second largest industry in this

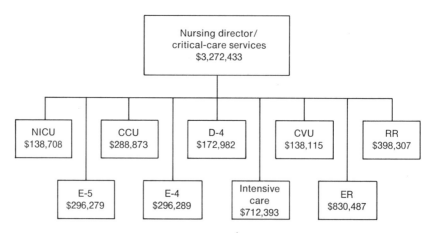

Fig. 3-1. Example of actual budget for each unit in critical-care service.

country. Health care costs have been increasing at an annual rate of 15%, which is approximately twice that of the general cost of living.

Because of the increase in the size of the health care industry as well as the inflationary effects of the costs of care, much national and state attention has been directed to health care. Many proposals have been and are being made to foster cost containment in health care. Pressures to control costs are being exerted by many sources such as consumer groups, health system agencies, state rate commissions, and the federal government. More recently, a 9% cap on hospital costs has been proposed; this trend is expected to continue.

What do all these developments mean for hospitals, directors of nursing, and critical-care unit directors? Plainly stated, we have come a long way in developing more sophisticated and accurate budgeting methods and procedures, but these techniques will seem simplistic when we experience what will occur over the next few years.

In the future, we can expect that standards of care will have to be delineated and followed before reimbursement will be received by the hospital. Third-party payors will examine even more closely the financial components that comprise the cost of patient. care. As the federal government becomes increasingly involved in financing the health care system, it will assume additional control. The possibility exists that in the future, patient care decisions will no longer be the sole responsibility of the physician. Approval for capital expenditures will be the first budget area curtailed because available funds will be limited.

It is strongly believed that standard cost systems will be developed within and among hospitals. Some states have already developed and are operating under uniform reporting systems. As these systems become more refined, each budgetary cost component will be more specifically delineated. When hospitals can more accurately identify costs and revenues, third-party payors will have to restructure their current inequitable reimbursement procedures.

Sophistication and refinement of budgetary processes is mandatory for the entire health care system. It will be necessary for critical-care unit directors as well as hospital and nursing administrators to learn the techniques to meet this challenge.

REFERENCES

1. Marriner, A.: Budgets, Superv. Nurse 8(4):53-56, 1977.
2. Ganong, J. M., and Ganong, W. L.: Nursing management, Germantown, Md., 1976, Aspen Systems Corporation.

BIBLIOGRAPHY

Carter unveils hospital payment "Cap" bill, vigorous opposition from health field vowed, Hospitals 51(10):17-19, 1977.

Freeman, G.: Profit planning and budgeting, Chief executive's handbook, Homewood, Ill., 1976, Dow Jones-Irwin, Inc.

Ganong, J. M., and Ganong, W. L.: Nursing management, Germantown, Md., 1976, Aspen Systems Corporation.

Gross, M. J.: Financial and accounting guide for nonprofit organizations, ed. 2, New York, 1974, Ronald Press.

Hawkins, B.: Nature of and reasons for cost increases under scrutiny, Hospitals **51**(7):113-116, 1977.

Marriner, A.: Budgets, Superv. Nurse **8**(4):53-56, 1977.

Mills, R.: A simple method for predicting days of increased patient census, J. Nurs. Adm. **7**(2):15-20, 1977.

Newmark, G. L.: Can quality be equated with cost? Hospitals **50**(7):81-86, 1976.

Schulz, R., and Johnson, A. C.: Management of Hospitals, New York, 1976, McGraw-Hill Book Co.

Slater, S. D.: The strategy of cash, New York, 1974, John Wiley & Sons, Inc.

Stevens, B. J.: What is the executive's role in budgeting for her department?, Hospitals **50**(22):83-86, 1976.

Zegeer, L. J.: Calculating a nurse staffing budget for a 20 bed unit at 100 per cent occupancy, J. Nurs. Adm. **7**(2):11-14, 1977.

DESIGNING AND EQUIPPING THE FACILITY

Health care facility construction has become a highly specialized field. This is due in part to the rapidly increasing technology that requires specific structural and utility components. The myriad of local, state, and federal regulations pertaining to hospital construction must be obeyed to the letter if a building project is to be completed. With the increase in rules, regulations, and complexity has come a dramatic rise in construction costs. Every effort should be made to accomplish well-thought out construction goals while containing costs whenever possible. In Chapter 4 Judith Thams has provided a step-by-step guide for the construction of a critical-care center with systems for determining the cost of various choices.

All future decisions depend on the ultimate purpose of the unit. It is ill-advised to embark on a critical-care building project without first defining the patient population to be cared for and collecting the data to determine the anticipated patient census for that particular disease. It is also necessary to survey the existing available facilities in which this type of patient problem is being treated. Hopefully the era of empire building is over, and the building of future facilities will be based on demographic data rather than political influence. When a well-documented determination of patient numbers and types of illnesses to be treated has been established, decisions concerning space, equipment, policies, and procedures follow. Each step in the planning process must be agreed on by hospital administration, the medical departments involved, and the nursing department. All three must have compatible expectations of the critical-care unit, or continual friction and disastrous misunderstandings will exist.

Every detail of the development, construction, and operation of a critical-care unit should be a team effort. The members and size of the team will change from one phase to the next, but at no time should the project be left to one or two people. Thams and Leslie K. Sampson (Chapter 5) have repeatedly emphasized the team concept in the design and construction of critical-care units. This idea brings attention to a deficiency of the past, since the input of nursing and ancillary service personnel has been ignored or overlooked in many hospital building projects. For a critical-care unit design and construction to be efficient and effective, personnel from all services involved in the operating aspect must be given the opportunity to contribute ideas.

Several designs of critical-care units are included as examples. The choice of a design may depend on the space available for construction or existing buildings. Each of the major configurations has advantages and disadvantages, and each has staunch advocates. To make a decision on building configuration, consult the architect, consider available space, visit units with the designs being considered, watch the nurses at work in the unit, talk with the paramedical personnel, and solicit the physicians' opinions. After collecting this information, a design compatible with unit needs can be chosen.

Perhaps more important than the overall design is attending to details that will change the unit from average to exceptional. Sampson has described many of these details, such as traffic patterns, acoustical considerations, lighting, and space allotments. The concept of the perimeter corridor holds a great deal of promise for reduction of traffic, noise, and contamination, but it can be difficult to implement unless there are no design constraints. When no other buildings, streets, access ways, and utility lines need be considered innovation can be exercised to the fullest. Most people today accept the concept of office space, classrooms, and lounge areas as part of the critical-care unit, but what a difference it makes if the office has a window, bright colors, and truly adequate space! Too many lounges are furnished with uncomfortable hand-me-downs instead of color-coordinated sofas and chairs purchased specifically for the area. A cheerful fully-equipped staff kitchen is a great staff morale booster.

James A. Van Drimmelen (Chapter 6) has presented the concept of materials handling in the hospital by applying industrial methods. The modular system is an idea whose time has come. Although the cost of conversion from outdated supply techniques to a modular method will preclude many hospitals from adopting the newer method, the modular system is ideal for facilities to be constructed in the future and for existing facilities that can afford the conversion. We have lived with the clutter of unplanned supplies stacked in every available spot long enough. The methods and choices to eliminate this problem are well-outlined in Van Drimmelen's chapter.

CHAPTER 4

Designing and developing
the critical-care unit

Judith Thams

Over the last 15 years, technology in hospitals has rapidly expanded in complexity. A significant amount of this growth has occurred in developing and improving critical-care medicine. The wide variety of equipment and procedures developed for the care of critically ill patients has created the need for highly sophisticated and complex facilities.

Because of this complexity, the design and development of critical-care units has become an important process that should be carefully undertaken to assure maximum flexibility and effectiveness once the unit is completed. For every dollar spent in construction of the facility, at least one dollar will be spent each year in operational costs. Therefore, investment of time and effort in the design process can save a significant amount of money and personnel frustration in operating the unit.

THE SYSTEMS ENGINEERING DESIGN METHODOLOGY

The design methodology suggested has been used in other industries and the military for many years. It is the systems engineering methodology, which is a team approach drawing on expertise from many disciplines to solve a complex problem (Fig. 4-1). The seven phases of this process as applied in industry are (1) initiation of the project, (2) organization of the primary team, (3) preliminary design, (4) principal design, (5) prototype construction, (6) test and training, and (7) production or implementation.[1]

Initiation

Initiation of the project may occur in many ways. This phase is simply the recognition of the need to undertake the project and a preliminary approval to proceed. Included are a definition of the problem, several suggested general

33

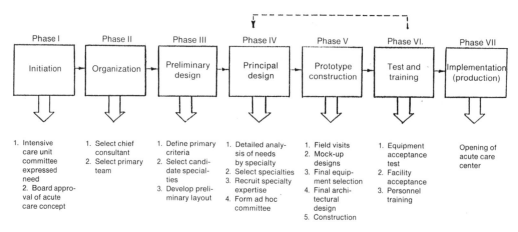

Fig. 4-1. A systems engineering model. (Modified from Goode, H., and Machol, R.: Systems engineering, New York, 1957, McGraw-Hill Book Co.)

sets of solutions, a statement of the types and numbers of team members needed, and a rough estimate of time and money needed.

The definition of the problem should be specific to provide a framework for the team to derive a solution. In addition, the problem statement should include overall goals and objectives, both in terms of facility design criteria and operational criteria.

The several suggested sets of solutions may involve preliminary evaluations for remodeling, relocating, or new construction.

A preliminary estimate is made of the types and numbers of team members needed. Consideration should be given to including a wide variety of team members at different phases of the design process. Although many hospitals do not have on staff all the expertise that would be required, consultants can and should be used to fill these gaps. The specialists to be considered are biomedical electronics and safety, infection control, industrial engineering, acoustics, construction management, and specialists in each of the medical and nursing specialties using the unit. Inclusion of these specialists should be emphasized because they assist in avoiding mistakes, the cost of which would far exceed the expense of the consultants.

Organization

This phase of design involves the selection of the key primary team members. These team members will head the project throughout the design phases. The team should be small and include, but not be limited to, a physician specializing in critical-care medicine, the critical-care nurse directly responsible for the unit(s), the project's chief architect, and an industrial engineer knowledgeable in systems engineering.

Large hospitals usually have the medical and nursing expertise necessary for designing a critical-care center. In many smaller hospitals this may not be the case. However, consultants knowledgeable in critical-care design can usually be found in a nearby university or teaching hospital if not available from within the institution. In one such case, the chairman of the ICU committee was selected as the project director, and another specialist was recruited from the university to assist the design team.

The primary task of the team in this phase is to develop a clear and concise problem statement and select a solution from the initial ones developed in the initiation phase. This solution will include such decisions as remodeling versus new construction, unit location, size of unit, and necessary support facilities.

Preliminary design

The preliminary design phase will result in a first version of the system. The team must refine and finalize the primary design and operational criteria in this phase.[2] These criteria include items such as (1) development of one critical-care center to include all specialties or separate independent units, (2) shared nursing staffs and nursing rotation through units or fixed nursing staffs, (3) physician staffing and organization, and (4) organizational and operational relationships with other departments.

If a large critical-care unit is to be developed with subdivided specialty areas, the criteria for each specialty area must also be finalized. For example, a center may include a burn unit, a respiratory unit, a surgical unit, and a medical unit within one complex.

Based on the established criteria, a preliminary layout is developed by the architect. This layout should be reviewed by all team members and several iterations may be necessary to achieve the objectives. In addition, trade-off studies may have to be made regarding the capability of meeting all criteria versus the constraints of money, land availability, or compromises imposed by remodeling an existing facility. Prior to finalizing the preliminary plans, the team should be expanded to assure appropriate design for the function intended.

Principal design

This phase consists of refining all design criteria so that the set of architectural plans can be developed. It will result in a final set of specifications from which the facility will be built.

It is important in this phase to include all team members, not only consultants but members of other hospital departments as well. Radiology, respiratory therapy, the pharmacy, and central services, to mention a few, can provide significant input to the design. Since these departments will be working with the critical-care unit(s), it is important to include them in reviewing the impact of their activities on the design.

At this time, the team may have become large enough to require formation of ad hoc committees to handle specific problems. For example, one group may evaluate and select equipment, whereas another may detail the design of the back panel at the head of the bed.

It is vitally important at this stage to include first-line supervisors who will be responsible for making the unit function and those who will supply services to the unit. Frequently, these people are aware of serious problems in the existing facility and can assist in avoiding the same or similar errors in the new facility.

Prototype construction

The last phase of the process is prototype construction, which can only be partially applied to hospitals. In industry, the resulting system will be constructed and used for tests and training. Based on the test procedures, suggested corrections or problems with the system will be referred back to the principal design team to correct any design deficiencies.

It is obvious that hospitals cannot afford to build a prototype and then go back to redesign. To accomplish the objectives of this phase, field visits to other critical-care units should be made. Discussion with personnel from units with similar equipment or design features can form the basis for acceptability and workability of the system.

In addition, mock-up of portions of the design such as the back panel design at the head of the bed can be developed without significant expense. In one project, a unit was being designed in an empty, shelled-in floor, and the floor plan was laid out with masking tape. This provided the team with a visual, full-scale layout to evaluate.

Test and training

Once construction is completed, the equipment should be tested, especially critical items such as monitors, oxygen, suction, and air. In a large unit, all items critical to patient safety are tested, whereas less important features may be tested on a random sampling basis. If items are found not to be in conformance with the specifications, the vendor should be called in to test these items and repair them prior to opening the unit.

The final phase of this step is instructing the personnel in equipment use. Other educational programs in policies and procedures should have been completed by this stage.

Implementation

In industry, this phase would encompass the mass production of the system. Because the process is modified to meet the needs of a hospital, this phase is the actual opening and use of the critical-care unit.

IDENTIFYING THE ARCHITECTURAL FIRM

One of the key team members will be the architect who must translate the criteria into a facility design and guide the project through construction. Frequently in hospital construction, the architect is selected by the administration and the Board of Directors. The architect is given general criteria on the budget and size of departments and then designs the facility with limited input from the hospital departments. The result is usually a design that is far from operationally ideal for the people who must care for patients in the facility. Because of the architect's key role in the design team, special emphasis must be placed on the selection of the architectural firm.

Certain basic steps should be taken even before actually approaching candidate firms so as to eliminate misunderstandings and to be certain to get off to a good relationship with a key person in your venture.

First, it is imperative that the persons who are to deal with the architect have a good understanding of the architect's role, capabilities, and limitations. Basically, the architect is your consultant on construction of your building, but provides services that are a good deal more. The architect's training and expertise will guide you not only through the entire physical building process, but also through the often complex legal aspects as well. In each of the fifty states, life, health, and safety are safeguarded through specific regulations or building codes. The drawings for new buildings or alterations to existing facilities must be approved by a licensed architect to assure inclusion of these regulations. In addition, the codes for hospitals are far more complex than for almost any other type of building. Therefore, an architect with experience in hospital work may be preferred.

A major factor in the selection of an architectural firm is the size of the project. A complex project may require a larger architectural firm. Large firms may have more manpower, resources, and experience and therefore are better qualified to handle the large complex projects. Smaller firms may, however, compensate for lack of experience with eagerness and creativity. It is not unusual for several small firms to work together on complex projects.

Consideration must be given to the proximity of the architect's office to the hospital's offices. During the design process frequent communication is required. If the architects are located in a distant city, this communication process can be greatly impeded. A local firm is usually more familiar with local conditions and codes.

Based on the determination of size of firm and locale, a list can be generated of firms who meet the criteria. The local chapter of the American Institute of Architects can provide a list of firms who meet the criteria and who would be interested in your type of project.

Individual meetings of the primary team and the prospective architectural firm will provide an opportunity to further learn of the architect's experience in design of critical-care units and capability to handle the job and complete the project within a specified time frame. It is also a time to meet the architect who would be in charge of the project. Ease of communication between the project architect and the team is essential to the success of the design.

Each firm should supply a complete list of facilities designed by the firm and specifically by the primary project architect along with a list of names of people in the facility who were responsible for the project.

Site visits to these facilities should be scheduled. Interviews should be conducted with as many of the persons who were involved in the project as possible. The important factors to determine from this visit are the architect's willingness and ability to communicate with the hospital personnel, the design criteria and how problems were solved, the client's satisfaction with the design solution, and unusual restrictions that may have been placed on the architect, which would have hindered the outcome of the solution. Although the resulting design may not be your ideal, you are trying to determine the architect's performance against the client's specific criteria and restrictions.

Once the architect is chosen, one team member should be appointed to coordinate all hospital activities with the architect. This person will be responsible for the flow of information between the in-house team members and the architect at each step of the process. Early in the process, the architect and other team members will work extensively together; this activity will taper off as the design approaches the solution. The architect will spend more time on structural, mechanical, and electrical details, whereas the rest of the team will concentrate on equipment. It is important, however, to keep the architect informed of equipment details that could affect the design. In addition, this person provides the architect with one in-house person responsible for resolving problems or conflicts.

IDENTIFYING THE LOCATION OF THE UNIT
Rationale for choice

An orderly approach should be maintained in selecting the proper location of the unit. Several choices may come to mind initially and should be evaluated so as to home in on the optimum area. Practical matters such as economics, pressing schedules, and unused space may, for example, quickly determine that new construction is out of the question and that remodeling of existing facilities is the only logical choice, or lack of space forces new construction. In most cases, however, the choice may not be so readily discerned, and a detailed study should be undertaken to arrive at a meaningful decision. Typically, a trade-off study is made to evaluate the many ramifications associated with the alternatives.

The initial step in the process is to complete a proximity chart (Fig. 4-2). The chart provides a basis for ranking the relationships of departments to each other. These relationships are divided into four categories: (1) necessary, the two areas must be close to one another; (2) desirable, barring other unforeseen problems, the areas should be adjacent; (3) unimportant; and (4) undesirable, because of traffic patterns, noise, sterile conditions, or other factors, the two areas should definitely not be adjacent.

The chart is completed by entering the appropriate value at the intersecting box for each two areas. For example, it may not be desirable to locate the

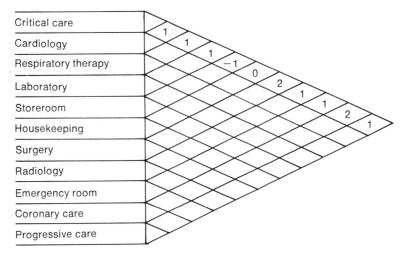

VALUES

VALUES

2 = desirable (the two areas
must be close to one another)

1 = desirable

0 = Unimportant

−1 = Undesirable (the two areas
should be separated from one another)

Fig. 4-2. Proximity chart permits ranking of departmental relationships.

critical-care area adjacent to the storeroom. Therefore, the intercept box shows a value of −1. On the other hand, it may be highly desirable to locate the critical-care unit adjacent to surgery: the intercept box shows a value of 2.

This chart will provide the basic data for the balance of the decision process. The form may be completed by several individuals within the organization. When values vary between people, a general consensus should be obtained from all primary design team members.

Some factors to be considered in developing a proximity chart include the following:

1. Moving the patient. If a special procedure room is not available or economically feasible within the critical-care area, frequent moves to other areas not only increase the risk to the patient, but may also require a critical-care nurse to accompany the patient. The long-term impact affects staffing levels and costs.

2. Medical staff backup. In smaller units, full-time medical coverage may not be feasible. Close proximity to the emergency room with 24-hour, physician coverage provides an opportunity for the emergency room physician to assist the critical-care unit in an emergency situation.

3. Staffing flexibility. If the critical-care unit is located adjacent to the coronary care unit (CCU) (if a separate CCU exists), the staff of each unit can provide backup to each other in an emergency or when staffing shortages exist in one unit but not in the other.

4. Transportation of equipment and supplies. Consideration must be given to the time required to transport both equipment and supplies to the unit, especially those items required in emergencies. Although it is desirable to have most items used in an emergency available within the unit, the cost of some items such as a portable x-ray machine, may prohibit this in smaller units or hospitals. In addition, it is preferable that the location chosen provide easy delivery of supplies without having to traverse the interior of the unit if at all possible.

Remodeling versus new construction

The next step in the trade-off study is to evaluate new construction versus remodeling if the change involves an existing facility. The numerous factors used in this portion of the evaluation are usually more readily quantified than those used in determining the rationale for location. For example, the cost of purchasing new property or for relocating existing departments may be obtained with some finite accuracy. In purchasing new property, the value of adjacent land may be already known from real estate sources, and the expense in connection with relocation of various units may be obtained from the architect.

The factors for remodeling or new construction include both physical and operational considerations.

Space availability. The initial evaluation should start with an analysis of available space. Consideration should first be given to areas with low-use services that might be eliminated because the need for them has changed or to any existing shelled-in space. Consideration should be given to the shape and constraint of the structure as well as total square footage to accommodate the necessary requirements for a critical-care area. Preliminary plans can be developed for the areas that would be adequate and cost estimates developed based on preliminary plans.

The next step is the evaluation of new construction. Alternate locations based on the proximity chart can be developed, and preliminary plans drawn. Again, cost estimates are developed for the new construction preliminary plans.

Use of old space. If the current space occupied by the critical-care area is required for other functions, a higher priority might be given to relocation rather than remodeling within the current area. In one case study, an open area seven-bed, intensive care unit with a two-bed isolation area was converted with minimal cost to a pediatric unit. The area provided good observation of the children and a large central play area readily visible from all points in the unit. The isolation rooms were used for isolation or separation of older children.

Disruptions to current operations. This factor is signficant to the critical-care area when remodeling of an existing unit or an area adjacent to an existing unit is being considered. To remodel an existing area means shutting down a portion or all of the unit. High demand for critical-care beds could eliminate the possibility of remodeling an existing area. In remodeling an adjacent area, noise factors may be a significant problem.

Maintaining revenue and operations. Closing a unit for remodeling or expansion could mean a loss of revenue as well as a threat to patient care. Estimates of loss of revenue can be developed and used in the analysis.

Conversion time. Conversion time becomes a critical factor, especially when demand for beds is high.

Adequate area for unit design. Especially in remodeling an existing space, consideration must be given to the amount of space required for the unit and for ancillary personnel. For example, the farther the unit is from respiratory therapy or the laboratory, the greater the need for a stat laboratory and respirator storage within the unit.

The need for future growth. Consideration must be given to the need for additional critical-care beds or additional support space in the future. Emphasis should be placed on achieving needed future expansion with a minimum of disruption to the planned unit.

Future hospital growth. Future overall hospital gowth must be considered in planning a facility. Care must be taken to place the unit so that it will not totally block growth of other very costly facilities such as radiology or surgery units.

Analysis of factors

A method for combining subjective and objective factors is used to arrive at an overall best solution from the trade-off study. The costs for each alternative are based on factors previously discussed and the preliminary plans. Table 1 lists the cost items to be considered for remodeling and new construction. All feasible alternatives should be considered.

The next step is the development of weighting factors for items that are not objectively quantifiable. Table 2 illustrates how to convert the proximity relationships to an overall weighting factor for two alternative plans. The desirability factors are listed as developed in Fig. 4-2 for the ideal proximities. Since no design may meet all these criteria, a method must be used to determine the most desirable location. In addition, proximity to one area may be more desirable than proximity to another area. To give one area a higher value than another, a weighting factor is developed (third column in Table 2).

Relative percentage values are developed so that the total of this column adds up to 100%. In Table 2 the values show that although it is desirable to have the critical-care area adjacent to both respiratory therapy and the laboratory, it is twice as important to be near the laboratory (10%) than respiratory therapy (5%). In addition, it is four times more important to be near

Table 1. Economic considerations of new construction versus remodeling

Alternative A		Alternative B	
New construction	**$**	**Remodeling**	**$**
Purchase of additional property and land preparation		Relocation costs of services in area	
Remodel existing building to tie into new construction		Demolition costs	
Additions to utilities to support new additions		Costs of downtime for services being relocated	
Demolition of unusable buildings		Remodeling costs	
Construction costs		Cost of lost revenue of unit	
Landscaping costs		Equipment costs	
Equipment costs	_____		_____
TOTAL COST		TOTAL COST	

Table 2. Weighting factors for proximity

Proximity of critical-care unit to	Desirability value*	Weight (%)	Alternative rating	
			Plan A	**Plan B**
Cardiology department	1	5	8	6
Respiratory therapy	1	5	7	9
Laboratory	1	10	10	5
Storeroom	−1	2	10	5
Housekeeping	0	2	5	5
Surgery	2	20	5	10
Radiology	1	15	8	6
Emergency room	1	15	6	4
Coronary care unit	2	20	10	8
Pulmonary care unit	1	6	8	6
Weighting factor		100	5.96	6.81
Weighting factor rounded off			6.00	7.00

*From Fig. 4-2.

Surgery (20%) than near the cardiology department (5%). These desirability and weighting factors are only examples. The actual values must be developed from the philosophies of each hospital and its medical staff.

Alternative rating values for each design must then be developed. The values are based on numbers from one to ten with ten being the best value. In the example, it is desirable for the laboratory to be near the critical-care area but not necessarily immediately adjacent to it. In the alternate ratings, it shows that the laboratory in Plan A is as close as desirable, but in Plan B it is not as close as it should be to the unit. Surgery is properly located in Plan B but its location is not as good in Plan A.

An overall weighting factor for each plan is developed by multiplying the

Table 3. Overall weighting factor

| | | Alternate ratings | | | |
| | | Plan A | | Plan B | |
	Weight* (%)	Rating	$ in 1,000	Rating	$
Proximity	20	6		7	
Space availability	4	9		6	
Use of vacated space	5	10		5	
Disruption to operations	10	1	100	10	0
Maintaining revenue and operations	10	2	500	10	0
Conversion time	6	8		6	
Overall unit design	20	5		8	
Future unit growth	10	2		10	
Future hospital growth	15	4		8	
Total construction costs			600		1,500
TOTAL	100	4.64*	$1,200	6.25	$1,500
Dollars/unit of weight			$ 258†		$ 240

*Weighting factor is weight × rating.
†Total dollars ÷ weighting factor.

percent weight, converted to a decimal value, by the rating for each factor, and adding the results. For Plan A the weighting factor is $(.05 \times 8) + (.05 \times 7) + (.10 \times 10) + (. . .) = 5.96$.

Based on these calculations, the alternative Plan B is more satisfactory in relationship to overall proximity with other departments than Plan A, since it resulted in a higher overall weighting factor.

The identical procedure is followed for each factor listed in this chapter. An overall value may be assigned to a factor or it may be evaluated in more detail as shown with the proximity factor. The values in Table 3 are only an example of the process. At this stage in the process, dollar values are used where appropriate. In this example Plan A might be a remodel of existing area, and Plan B would be for new construction. Therefore, Plan A shows a dollar value of $100,000 in costs because of disruption to operations and $500,000 in lost revenue because of the need to close part of the unit. The rating values are also signficantly lower because of the patient care impact of closing part of the unit and disruption to operations. In Plan B, the unit is not disrupted, revenue is not lost, and the plan has no impact on patient care.

The final step in the trade-off study is to compare the total cost to the weight. The total dollars are divided by the weighting factor to obtain a dollar value for each unit of weight. In the example in Table 3, the remodel cost (Plan A) is less than the new construction plan (Plan B). The dollar cost for each unit of weight to achieve a better design is less, therefore, Plan B would be more desirable.

This example is obviously an extreme case; not all alternatives might have such dramatic differences. However, the methodology described in this chapter provides a mechanism for formally evaluating numerous trade-offs and comparing design factors to costs.

CHOOSING THE FLOOR PLAN

The overall plan of the critical-care area is frequently restricted by the general shape and configuration of the hospital and the ideal location selected for the unit. Any floor plan may have some drawbacks; however, the planning process attempts to minimize the number and severity of drawbacks and maximize the use of the design. The total square footage required will equal approximately two and one half to three times the bed space.

Traffic patterns

Traffic patterns include movement of patients, personnel, supplies, equipment, and visitors. Criteria for each category should be considered separately.

Transportation patterns of patients to and from the unit should ideally be separated from public corridors and visitor waiting areas. If patient transport requires elevators, a separate oversized elevator should be designated for this purpose.

The unit design should provide storage for equipment and clean and dirty supplies in a location near the nurses' station, preferably off an exterior corridor so that personnel stocking the supplies do not have to enter the unit.

The nurses' station, medication area, and supply areas should be centrally located within the unit to reduce personnel travel distances as much as possible.

The visitor's access to the unit should be visible from the nursing station to facilitate visitor control.

Patient room

The design of the patient rooms should provide optimal surveillance from the nurses' station as well as access to the patient. Ideally, all patients should be clearly visible from the nursing station; however, in larger units, visibility from other patient areas may suffice for a few beds, since the majority of nursing activity is at the bedside rather than the nursing station.

The open patient room is far more efficient in terms of space use and nursing care. One of the main disadvantages of large, open patient care areas is the noise level. To achieve the benefits of the open area and reduce the noise factor, beds can be grouped in twos or threes. The open area between the beds provides shared space for large equipment, and the walls reduce the noise between the bays. In addition, one nurse can have easy access to both patients.

The ideal bed orientation is perpendicular to the exterior wall, or the foot of the bed toward the nursing station. Immediate access to both sides of the bed is provided, and the nurses have full vision of the patients' faces. The only disadvantage is that patients do not have a window view, since they face away from the exterior wall. When the bed orientation is parallel to the exterior wall, nursing visibility of the patients' face is reduced. In addition, a large area is required for the same degree of access to both sides of the bed.

Isolation rooms should have private baths and an anteroom for gowning, masking, and handwashing. These rooms should be located so that dirty items being removed from rooms are not transported past other open bed areas. Both forward and reverse airflow should be provided. Room use will be improved if the interior wall is a large sliding glass door that can be opened for nonisolated patients.

The minimum sizes of rooms will vary with the design. An open area should contain a minimum of 150 square feet for each bed, a closed room a minimum of 175 to 200 square feet for each bed, and an isolation room should have a minimum of 225 to 250 square feet for each bed.

Sinks for handwashing should be provided in each private room or one sink for every two beds in an open area.

Nursing station

The nursing station should be centrally located with visibility over the counters to all patient areas. The monitoring area should include an area for the ward clerks to work. This allows the ward clerk to activate the strip chart recorder when irregularities occur on the monitors that nurses would not see when working at the bedside. Charting space for several nurses should be provided even in a small unit. An area should be provided for physicians to chart, and a separate cubicle near the station for physicians to dictate. A sink should be provided near the nurses' station for handwashing.

It is recommended that a separate room adjacent to the nurses' station be provided for preparing medications. The area should be glass on one side, so that the nurse may maintain visual contact within the unit.

Support areas

Additional areas within or immediately adjacent to the unit are required for the functioning of a critical-care unit. These areas are the ones most frequently overlooked when not required by building codes.

Hospital building codes require areas for clean and soiled utility and linen. The soiled utility room should have a sink and a hopper. In addition, a separate room should be provided for storage of equipment such as bed scales and ventilators. This room should have numerous electrical outlets, since much of the critical-care equipment is battery-operated and needs to be recharged while stored.

A small stat laboratory should be available within the area, if the main laboratory is not in close proximity. A special procedures room is highly desirable within the immediate vicinity, but may only be economically feasible with larger units (over eight beds). A conference room should be available in the unit for physicians and nurses.

Even in small units, a physician lounge should be immediately adjacent to the unit. In larger units, sleeping cubicles off the physician lounge provide separate sleeping areas for a resident or staff physician.

A toilet for nursing personnel should be available in the unit, with a lounge area immediately adjacent to the unit supplied with lockers and coat racks.

If the unit has a medical director, an office should be provided for the director with space for a secretary.

Large units will require an office for the nursing supervisor and clinical nurse specialists for the unit. Space for storage of educational materials (tests and audiovisual equipment) and reference materials should be provided either in the office area or in a nearby classroom if the conference room is not large enough for clinical teaching.

Public areas

A large comfortable waiting area for family should be adjacent to the critical-care area. An average of two seats for each bed should be provided for up to twelve beds. For more than twelve beds, an average of one and one half seats for each bed would be adequate. The room should be furnished in warm colors with carpeting, television, radio, and an in-house telephone restricted to incoming calls for people trying to contact family at the hospital. Public telephones should be available immediately outside the waiting room for visitors to make outside calls. Public restrooms should be adjacent to the waiting room. Ideally, small cubicles in which family members can sleep should be provided. Although most hospitals discourage family members from spending the night at the hospital, some will insist. The cubicles can also double as consulting rooms for the physician to meet with the family.

If the waiting room is not large enough to divide into a smoking and nonsmoking area, good air circulation should be provided, or smoking should be prohibited.

Typical floor plan

Several typical floor plans are presented in this section to demonstrate the advantages and disadvantages of different designs. Fig. 4-3 is a detailed floor plan for a multidisciplinary critical-care center developed at a west coast facility. The plan used an existing shelled-in floor to incorporate four eight-bed units with a central core support area. The medical/surgical and pulmonary ICUs featured open bay areas (12 feet by 14 feet) with two isolation rooms (15 feet by 15 feet each), and the coronary and progressive ICUs were designed with private rooms (12 feet by 14 feet for each bed). The detailed design of each patient area is identical so that a nurse could work in any unit and always be familiar with the layout.

The unit includes built-in defibrillators and drawers for emergency drugs

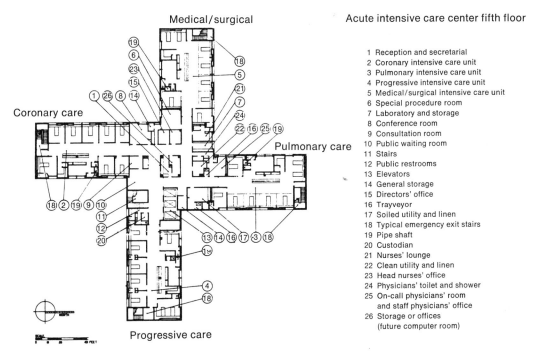

Medical/surgical

Acute intensive care center fifth floor

1 Reception and secretarial
2 Coronary intensive care unit
3 Pulmonary intensive care unit
4 Progressive intensive care unit
5 Medical/surgical intensive care unit
6 Special procedure room
7 Laboratory and storage
8 Conference room
9 Consultation room
10 Public waiting room
11 Stairs
12 Public restrooms
13 Elevators
14 General storage
15 Directors' office
16 Trayveyor
17 Soiled utility and linen
18 Typical emergency exit stairs
19 Pipe shaft
20 Custodian
21 Nurses' lounge
22 Clean utility and linen
23 Head nurses' office
24 Physicians' toilet and shower
25 On-call physicians' room
   and staff physicians' office
26 Storage or offices
   (future computer room)

Coronary care

Pulmonary care

Progressive care

Fig. 4-3. Detailed floor plan of existing critical-care center. (Courtesy Anaheim Memorial Hospital, Anaheim, Calif.)

and supplies at each patient bedside. The core area provides a family waiting area with a secretary to control visitor traffic, special procedures room, stat lab, conference room, consultation room, medical director's office, clean and soiled utility and linen rooms, nurses' lounge, on-call physician lounge, and computer room.

Limitations of the design were established by the existing shape of the building. The major limitation of this design was the core space; it should have been approximately 50% larger for the number of beds included. The waiting area contains 165 square feet and should have been a minimum of 300 square feet. Offices and storage space were not provided for the clinical nurse specialists, and an additional storage area is required for large equipment.

The other major drawback is that the center is located on the fifth floor, whereas the surgery and radiology department and the emergency room are located on the first floor. One elevator is assigned to patient transport to and from the unit and is not available to the public or employees.

Visibility of patients in the corner rooms from the nursing station is limited, but there is good visibility to these rooms from all other areas. However, advantages of the design are far more numerous and provide an excellent solution to restrictions of the existing building.

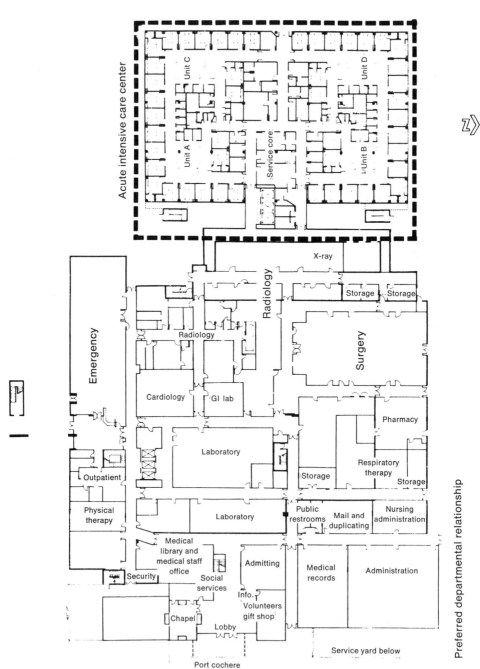

Fig. 4-4. Architect's plan for preferred location of new critical-care center. (Courtesy Anaheim Memorial Hospital, Anaheim, Calif.)

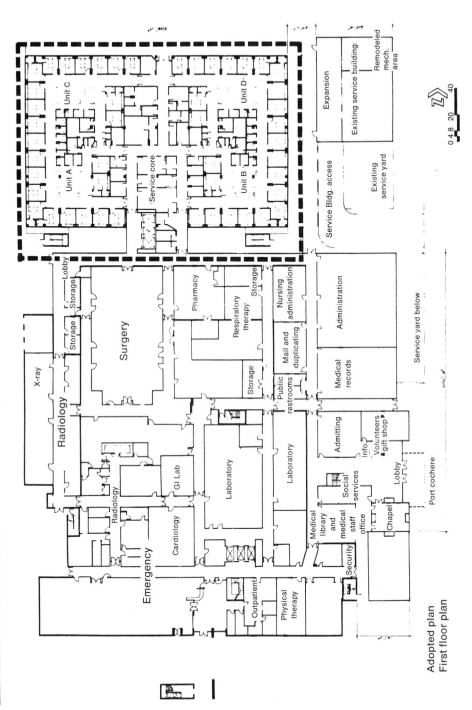

Fig. 4-5. Plan adopted for new critical-care center, which differs from preferred plan because of building constraints. (Courtesy Anaheim Memorial Hospital, Anaheim, Calif.)

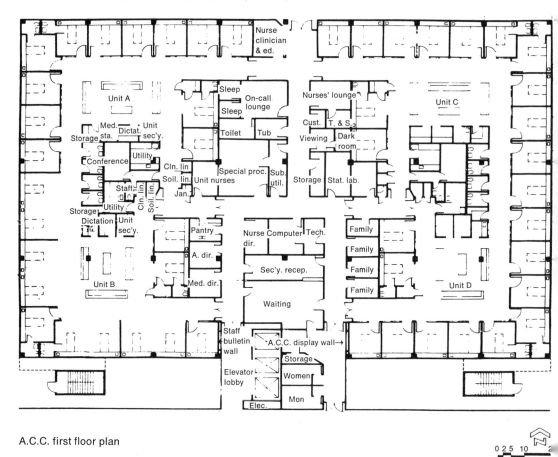

A.C.C. first floor plan

0 2 5 10

Fig. 4-6. Detailed floor plan of new critical-care center. (Courtesy Anaheim Memorial Hospital, Anaheim, Calif.)

Traffic patterns separate visitors from the activity of the center except during visiting hours. Support areas are centrally located and shared with four units. Patient rooms are large with good access. The open bay area is subdivided into two patient bed areas on the end and two isolation rooms.

An overall design, incorporating a large critical-care center in proximity to other departments, is illustrated in Fig. 4-4. In this design the critical-care unit is adjacent to the emergency room, surgery, and the radiology department. The actual final design is detailed in Fig. 4-5. The limitation was imposed by a medical office center that forced the critical-care center to be placed away from the emergency room. Lack of proximity to the emergency room can be compensated for, however, since the area has a paramedic system. Patients who are sufficiently stabilized by the paramedics can be directly admitted to the center.

The detailed design (Fig. 4-6) incorporates all the features previously discussed in this chapter. The unit combines private rooms for coronary and progressive care patients with two-bed open areas for medical/surgical care patients. Primary isolation rooms and large oversized rooms are provided in each corner for patients requiring dialysis or major equipment support such as a balloon pump.

The design provides two twelve-bed units back to back to allow for overlap of staff support between the units. A twelve-bed unit size was chosen because of staffing considerations. A unit clerk can be fully used in a twelve-bed unit but may not be fully used in a smaller unit. Nurse/patient ratios can be improved when unexpected staffing shortages occur. For example, an average nurse/patient ratio is 1:2 (12 hours for each patient day). An eight-bed unit would therefore require four nurses and a twelve-bed unit, six nurses. If the eight-bed unit is short one nurse a shift, the actual hours for each patient day are 9 hours. If the twelve-bed unit is short one nurse a shift, the actual hours for each patient day are 10 hours amounting to 1 hour for each patient more than in a smaller unit.

The design provides for supplying the unit without transversing the interior of the unit, removing soiled items from isolation without passing other bed areas, adequate support space within the unit, and ample core support area for the center.

REFERENCES

1. Goode, H., and Machol, R.: Systems engineering, New York, 1957, McGraw-Hill Book Co., pp. 35-45.
2. Thams, J. A., and Whipple, G. H.: Community hospital intensive care design, Industral Engineering **5**:32-39, May, 1973.

BIBLIOGRAPHY

Bobrow, M. L., and Craft, N. C.: Planning ICU and CCU facilities, Hospitals **45**:47-51, May 16, 1971.

Clipson, C. W., and Werber, J. J.: Planning for cardiac care, Ann Arbor, Mich., 1973, The Health Administration Press.

Manual of surgical intensive care, American College of Surgeons Committee on Pre- and Post-Operative Care, Philadelphia, 1977, W. B. Saunders Co.

Special care units, Mod. Hosp., pp. 81-99, Jan., 1972.

Weil, M. H., et al.: A new approach to critical care units, Hospitals **45**:65-68, Aug. 16, 1971.

Whipple, G. H.: Acute coronary care, Boston, 1972, Little, Brown & Co.

Wiklund, P. E.: Intensive care units: design, location, staffing ancillary areas, equipment, Anesthesiology **31**:122-136, Aug., 1969.

CHAPTER 5

Designing and equipping
the critical-care unit

Leslie K. Sampson

The physical and environmental design of these specialized units can either enhance or obstruct the effective use of human capabilities in critical care. The challenge of designing a unit that takes into account the human factors and requirements of both patients and hospital staff requires collaboration of architects, administrators, nurses, physicians, and technicians.

IDENTIFYING AN ARCHITECTURAL FIRM

Identifying an architectural firm with whom to collaborate on the unit design is an obvious first step. This decision should be made by a committee consisting of nurses, administrators, plant engineers, physicians, and staff from housekeeping. Potential firms that specialize in hospital design should be asked to submit sample designs of previous work and to provide a list of the location of facilities they have designed. The committee can conduct visits to these selected facilities to evaluate the effective use of space and design. Interviews with the staff working in these units can identify both the positive and problematic aspects of the unit from an experienced point of view.

The difficulties inherent in the project can be eased by effective communication between committee members and the architectural firm. Interviews with committee members from previously constructed facilities identify the extent of dialogue and responsiveness of the architect. After obtaining and reviewing a relevant data base on the design capabilities, experience, communication process, and responsiveness to expressed needs, an architectural firm can be selected.

IDENTIFYING THE UNIT LOCATION

Location of the unit should be identified next, and the many variables considered. Whether the unit is for a single health problem, such as a neonatal intensive care unit, or for multiple problems such as a medical/surgical intensive care unit, will greatly affect the final decision. The neonatal intensive care unit should obviously be located close to the delivery room, whereas the medical/surgical intensive care unit should be near step-down or progressive care areas and others with similar functions. For example, close proximity of allied units, such as an accident ward, ICU, operating suite, and recovery unit, can simplify the sharing of common facilities, equipment, and staff. Staff-sharing feasibility, advantages, and disadvantages should be reviewed in depth, and a basic policy established. Space requirements for progressive care areas adjacent to the critical-care area must be evaluated at this time, since it will affect selection of the final location. Although some units are windowless and are located centrally within the building, it is generally accepted that reality orientation is enhanced with windows, allowing observation of external activities and light changes.[1-3]

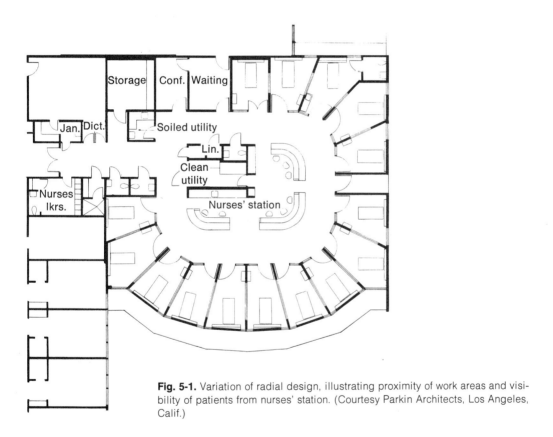

Fig. 5-1. Variation of radial design, illustrating proximity of work areas and visibility of patients from nurses' station. (Courtesy Parkin Architects, Los Angeles, Calif.)

Intensive care unit

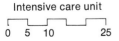

0   5   10   25

The institution's needs will generally determine if new construction or remodeling is to take place. Because of expanding critical-care technology with its complexity of concealed electrical and physiological signal wiring, gas distribution systems, and need to build monitoring hardware and life-support equipment in the patient bed area, remodeling of an existing unit may not be the most cost-effective method. In many hospitals, general care units have been converted into critical-care areas. This frequently has resulted in poor patient visibility, congested traffic patterns, inadequate space for bedside placement of monitoring hardware and life-support equipment, makeshift central monitoring stations, inadequate storage space for equipment and supplies, and insufficient conference and lounge facilities. An innovative facility designer can minimize trade-offs in the remodeling process if the planning team has communicated the critical-care unit requirements effectively. The greatest potential for successful integration of design criteria, which provides an optimal environment for the critical-care patient and efficient delivery of required care, exists in new construction with variations on a radial layout (Fig. 5-1). The radial layout allows observation of all patients from the central station and permits the design of a peripheral service corridor that reduces visitor and ancillary personnel traffic in patient areas. A separate service core with access to the staff work areas is another advantage. Nonetheless, design criteria to be considered include the floor plan, utility service systems, environmental features, equipment, and methods of stocking and supplying patient care materials.

FLOOR PLAN

The actual design of the unit will be the result of a complete analysis of many different factors. These factors will help establish requirements needed for the specific critical-care unit that, when communicated to the architect, will result in an optimal physical design.

Traffic patterns within the unit must be closely analyzed with specific attention to minimizing the possibility of conversational groups forming in open areas. This may be accomplished by providing centrally located enclosed conference/charting areas.

Travel distance to storage or supply areas should be minimized as well as the movement of visitors and ancillary services (central supply and linen delivery) through patient areas. An effective solution is to include a perimeter corridor providing direct access to patient rooms and utility and storage areas. This may not always be feasible when remodeling is chosen rather than new construction. However, a careful and detailed analysis of the placement of utility and storage areas and the resulting routes to patient rooms should be done to assure that the same objectives are met.

As previously mentioned, windows are beneficial for patient reality orientation. The placement of the unit should take into account natural illumination and view. The position of the patients' beds within the unit should allow a direct view of the window as well as a line of vision to the nursing central station (Fig. 5-2). The latter provides reassurance that a staff member is always available when help is needed and facilitates observation of the patient by the unit staff. Another consideration for windows is whether they should be permanently closed or have the capability of being opened. Since most critical-care units are air-conditioned and must have a state-specified number of air turnovers an hour, it would not seem necessary to have windows that open. Unfortunately, air conditioners do break down, fail to operate during power loss, and require periodic maintenance. Therefore, security-screened windows that open will provide ventilation and access to the outside when needed. In case of fire the windows will provide a means for the fire department to directly remove smoke.

Most states, the federal government, and the JCAH have published guidelines for special care units. These regulations must be carefully observed and incorporated during the planning stages. Since standards of care vary from hospital to hospital, the type and amount of equipment and the unit size and future requirements will be considerably different. Sufficient space

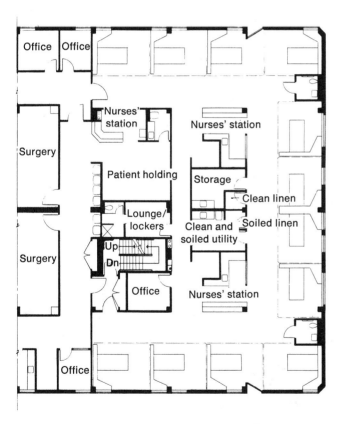

Cardiac care unit

```
0    5   10           25
```

Fig. 5-2. Critical-care unit adjacent to surgical suites permits each patient an outside window view, as well as visual contact with nurses' station. (Courtesy Parkin Architects, Los Angeles, Calif.)

for easy access to the patient must be provided, not only for the uncomplicated patient, but also for emergency care and the complex multisystem failure patient requiring several types of life-support equipment, treatment, and diagnostic and monitoring devices. Space requirements can be determined by the size and placement of the ventilator, monitor, transducers, etc. One method of providing complete access to the patient from all sides and ends of the beds is to have all electrical, gas, and vacuum outlets provided in a ceiling-hung or free-standing column positioned at one corner of the bed (Figs. 5-3 and 5-4). The bed may then be positioned several feet away from the head wall, permitting access to the patient from the head of the bed. Clearance for portable equipment, such as resuscitation carts, x-ray units, and electrocardiograph (ECG) machines, should be sufficient at the foot of the bed, even when the head of the bed is moved away from the head wall 24 inches, or when devices such as ventilators, hypothermia/hyperthermia units, and suction devices are required. Because of these needs, a critical-care patient's room should be 175 to 200 square feet in size[4]; an open bay-type unit should allow a minimum 150 square feet for each bed.

Within the patient area there must be space for storage of the patient's necessary personal items, supplies required for patient care (dressings, tape,

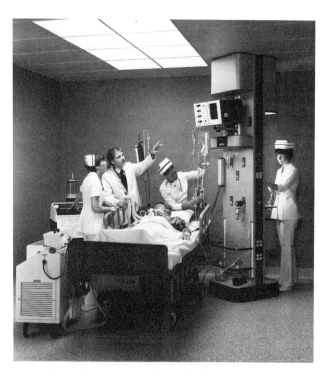

Fig. 5-3. Ceiling-hung supply column. (Courtesy Hill-Rom Company, Inc., Batesville, Ind.)

suction catheters, gloves, electrodes, etc.), linen, and bedpans. Bedside stands have traditionally served this purpose. Floor space can be freed by having storage units built into the wall. Bed tables must also be considered as space takers and may be stored out of the way in wall niches constructed for that purpose. In addition, the cluttered bedside stand and the bed table have done double duty as inefficient work surfaces, as have the tops of many electrial devices (a dangerous practice to be avoided) in the clinical area. Shelving constructed at the head of the bed provides an area for items such as trays, irrigation kits, and intravenous fluids. Seating can be provided for visitors by a flip-down seat attached to the wall.

If one accepts that the best method of preventing cross-contamination is

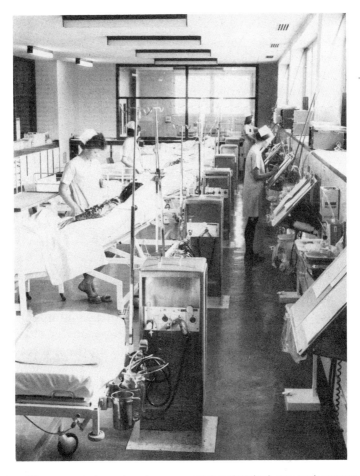

Fig. 5-4. Series of floor-mounted supply columns containing electrical, gas, and vacuum connections that permit access to head of patient's bed. (Courtesy Anthony Fisher, FFARCS, The Radcliffe Infirmary, Oxford, England.)

handwashing, then sinks deep and wide enough to prevent splashing and equipped with knee-operated faucets must be available in each room. Such provisions will encourage the practice of handwashing after caring for each patient and hopefully reduce nosocomial infections.

The central nurses' station should be placed exactly as the name suggests, centrally. Observation of and quick access to all patients from the nurses' station can be accomplished by the innovative architect who understands these requirements. Design criteria for the central station should include provision for adequate, comfortable charting space for the team members (nurses, physicians, respiratory and physical therapists, social workers, etc.). This charting area should be coordinated, but separate from the ward clerks' work area so that charts, forms, and stationery are available in one centralized area. In large units (more than twelve patients), a separate receptionist area at the unit entrance facilitates visitor control and communication functions.

The decision to use central monitoring depends on the unit purpose. It is generally accepted that coronary care units should have central monitoring. Unless central monitors are continually scanned by a knowledgeable staff member, their usefulness is questionable where computerized data retrieval does not exist. Central monitoring equipment should be placed where personnel can easily observe the patterns and the patients being monitored. To permit visualization of all patients in large units, the central nurses' station may have to be decentralized into two or more areas. Because larger units have increased numbers of staff, decentralization of the monitoring station will reduce the level of congestion in a single area.

If the unit or patient rooms are open to traffic and work areas, the central nurses' station may be enclosed with ceiling-high safety glass to afford conversational privacy for the staff and decrease the annoying intensities and sounds reaching the patients. This still permits visual observation of the patients by the nursing staff and reassures patients that staff members are present.

The medication area, when located in the central nurses' station, should be enclosed to permit preparation of patient medications with as little distraction and disturbance as possible. A comfortable, soundproof staff lounge with toilet facilities should be provided on the perimeter of the unit. Many staff members prefer to have breaks and meals in the critical-care area because of patient requirements, possible emergencies, and uniform policies. For this reason, the lounge should have a nourishment center with a refrigerator for keeping simple meals and beverages. Comfortable chairs and couches should be available to permit quiet relaxation. The lounge should have telephones and be connected to the emergency alarm and intercom systems. A secure locker room adjacent to the lounge will allow the staff to store personal articles. It may serve as a dressing room, should scrub attire be required for staff members providing direct patient care.

Continuing education activities, nurse and physician conferences and staff meetings are an everyday part of critical care and are facilitated by the immediate availability of a conference room. The unit conference room should be supplied with a chalkboard, film screen, x-ray viewer, conference table, chairs, and electrical outlets for audiovisual equipment. A locked closet or cabinet should be available in the room for equipment such as a tape recorder and 35 mm slide projector. A three- or four-shelf portable library cart that can also be used in the unit or lounge is suggested. If security is a problem, the books can be attached to the cart.

The visitors' lounge should provide ample comfortable seating for family and friends of the patients. To take the monotony out of waiting, it is desirable to have available a television or piped-in music and current magazines and books. Pay telephones must be nearby for visitors to communicate patient changes or individual needs to family members or others. Cubicles with fold-down cots may also be provided to permit visitors privacy and rest. Toilet and shower facilities should be accessible from the lounge and large enough to permit visitors to freshen up during long vigils. A smaller family room, available for private conferences between staff, clergy, and family members in crisis, will be frequently used.

If the institution requires that a physician be available in the unit 24 hours a day, an on-call sleep room with toilet and shower facilities should be included in the floor plan. A telephone and alarm system linked directly to the unit must be installed.

Utility rooms are best located within the critical-care unit, but access must be from within the unit and also from the hospital corridor, to facilitate removal and replacement of supplies. This reduces the traffic and noise in patient care areas. To prevent contamination of clean supplies, separate clean and dirty utility rooms are required with separate access doors. As many storage cabinets as possible should be provided but will, of course, depend on the space allocated, the shape of the room, and the door and/or window location. Space must be identified and allocated for storage of linen and central supply items needed for patient care. These items might be stored in cabinets, shelving, or on carts placed in the designated storage niche and exchanged daily.

To prevent equipment accumulation from cluttering work areas, patient care areas, and traffic pathways, a large storeroom is absolutely essential. Bulky items such as wheelchairs, stretchers, ECG machines, ventilators, hypothermia/hyperthermia units, gastric intermittent-suction machines, wheeled carts, scales, and commodes can only be secured out of sight when adequate storage is provided. The storage room must be spacious enough so that the equipment is readily available and easy to remove when needed. If adequate storage is not provided, the equipment will be stored in corridors, creating a fire hazard.

One of the most neglected areas in the design of critical-care areas is the housekeeping facilities. This separate room must include a disposal system for contaminated scrub or mop solutions as well as a clean water supply for preparing new solutions. Shelves for storing cleaning chemicals, hooks for hanging mops, etc., a bulletin board for solution-mixing instructions, and environmental control policies are required. Housekeeping personnel are an important but frequently overlooked part of the critical-care team. When unit culture reports are shared, emphasizing the vulnerability of the patient population, the need for meticulous cleaning is highlighted.

Adequate office space immediately adjacent to the unit should be available for the unit medical and nursing directors, secretary, and leadership staff. Storing unit data, records, and personnel files nearby will facilitate and permit a smoother functioning unit. Offices for the critical-care supervisory or managerial nurses and physicians located within the immediate vicinity of the unit permits greater visibility to the staff, makes possible observation of and consultation with the staff, allows a more active participation in clinical activities, and provides a closer identification with the unit.

Twenty-four–hour laboratory analysis is a requirement for the ICU. Satellite laboratories are a proven asset for large institutions where the time lag for delivery of specimens and reporting of results is dangerous and unacceptable. These satellite facilities can serve as stat laboratories for several units to increase their cost-effectiveness. Laboratory personnel should be as carefully screened for reliability and expertise as are the critical-care nursing staff members. Inclusion in patient rounds and conferences will increase their involvement with the patient's needs.

Some large institutions have found satellite pharmacies to be necessary. The pharmacist could provide formal and informal in-service sessions for drugs being introduced into the unit and make rounds with the nurse and physician to provide input as to the effectiveness, appropriateness, and compatibility of drugs being used or considered. Whether a satellite pharmacy exists or not, the benefits of having a regularly assigned pharmacist make daily rounds with the staff cannot be overemphasized.

CONSTRUCTION

Once the unit location and floor plans have been finalized, construction and remodeling requirements and costs need to be considered. An estimate would be expected to cover these phases as well as installation of air conditioners, lighting, electrical wiring, plumbing, pipe systems for compressed air, oxygen, and vacuum as well as conduit for monitoring system cables, intercommunication, and nurse call systems. The telephone company will charge a supplementary fee for telephone wiring and jack installation at each patient bed. To minimize a future need to expand or modify the construction, careful evaluation of past and current trends should be undertaken to predict likely requirements 10 years from the construction completion date.

Plumbing should service only the critical-care unit(s). Control valves must be installed on pipes entering the unit to allow service to be turned off, should breaks occur. This could prevent damage to the expensive and sophisticated electrical monitoring and life-support equipment.

Electrical service must be provided by a separate branch circuit, servicing only the critical-care unit(s). A supplemental emergency power source, which is connected by a feeder to an automatic switching device that will supply power to all electrical outlets within 10 seconds after interruption of the normal power source, is required at all patient care areas. Outlets connected to the emergency power source must be clearly identified. The circuit breaker panel for the patient care and work areas should be located within the unit. The nursing staff must have access to it, and the circuit breakers should be clearly labeled as to the location of the single duplex outlet each services. A minimum of ten grounded 110-volt electrical outlets should be located within a few feet of the patient's bed and placed approximately 36 inches above the floor to facilitate connection and discourage disconnecting the power plug from the outlet by pulling the power cord. In addition, a 220-volt outlet should be accessible to each room for portable x-ray equipment requiring this voltage level.

Telephone service for patients in critical-care units has often not been provided; however, many alert patients will benefit from being permitted to place telephone calls. Incoming calls, however, disturb seriously ill patients. Since incoming calls cannot be effectively monitored, they should not be allowed, which gives the patient the choice of whom and when to telephone. Telephone jacks installed near each bed and one or two portable phones stored in the nursing station are considered adequate. The phones may be taken to the patient's bedside when required.

Most critical-care patients will require ventilatory assistance, support, or therapy with supplemental humidified oxygen and/or compressed air. Both the main and reserve supply bank providing 50 pounds per square inch (psi) of compressed gas should be available to each critical-care bed area. Audible and visible alarms must be installed in the engineering work or office area and also in the critical-care nursing work area. Alarms indicate malfunctions in the system because of pressures deviating from preestablished ranges. Manual shutoff valves must be located and identified in both the engineering area and the critical-care unit to permit interruption of the supply by engineering or nursing personnel in case of fire, excessive pressure, or for repair purposes (Fig. 5-5). Minimally, one outlet for each compressed gas should be provided on each side of the bed approximately 5 feet above the floor. The outlets should be of an approved quick-coupling and noninterchangeable type[5] for one-handed connection and disconnection of the regulator-gauge assembly. They should be easy to clean, clearly labeled, and color coded for easy identification and safety. If the twist-lock, regulator-gauge assembly is used, the outlets should be placed 12 inches apart, center to center, to provide space for quick coupling with the humidifier attached.

A central vacuum system is preferable to portable bedside suction units. A vacuum is necessary for suctioning secretions from the pulmonary tract, providing continuous suction for chest and sump tubes, and for intermittent low-level gastrointestinal suction. The system should provide a vacuum level of 0

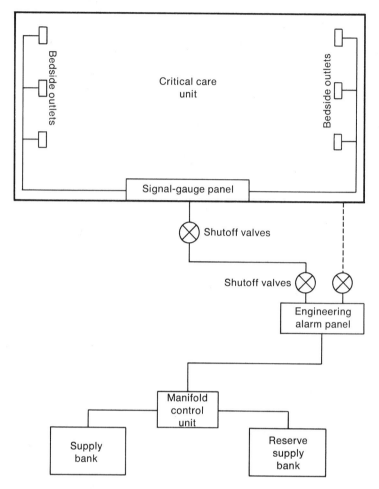

Fig. 5-5. Schematic drawing of oxygen system with supply, controls, and shut-off valves. Compressed air systems use compressor, and vacuum systems use vacuum pump in place of supply and reserve banks.

to 200 mm Hg at each outlet with alarm panels and manual shutoff valves located in a similar manner as required for compressed gases. A minimum of three outlets should be placed at the same level as the oxygen and compressed air outlets and spaced over both sides of the bed at least 12 inches away from other outlets. Vacuum outlets should also be of an approved[6] quick-coupling and noninterchangeable type, color coded and labeled, and easily cleaned. The collection containers must be firmly supported and protected from accidental damage caused by moving beds and other equipment.

ENVIRONMENTAL CONSIDERATIONS

Patients and staff alike are affected by the critical-care environment. A well-thought out and executed floor plan promotes efficiency and order; environmental decisions concerning visual interest, acoustics, illumination, thermal comfort, privacy, and safety will either enhance or weaken the best design. Whatever is chosen to enhance the patients' surroundings should be easy to clean and maintain.

The color scheme of the critical-care unit should be selected with as much care as the equipment. Much has been written about the effects of various colors on mankind. The color or colors selected should promote rest but not depress the patient and provide a calming but not boring effect on the staff. If a wall in the central station would lend itself to a mural or graphic design, it would provide visual interest.

Windows were discussed earlier as an important aspect of reality orientation for patients. Additional ways of orienting the patient are to provide an easily seen clock and a calendar showing only the day and date. A calendar/clock with a ceiling digital display of the day, date, and time would be ideal. A pillow speaker is useful in providing the date, day, time, music, and news. Portable battery-operated radios (without a battery charger) with earphones may also be used. Many patients in critical-care units will not be able to watch television, but it is a welcome distraction and time-consumer for coronary, burn, and transplant patients and others requiring critical care who are mentally alert and bored. Depending on the patient population, provision for television can be made at selected beds. Properly installed and maintained monitoring equipment will not be affected by television. Electrical hazards can be eliminated by placing the television out of reach, allowing patients to change channels by remote control or by using a battery-operated model (battery charger should not be used). The only valid factors, aside from cost, in considering the use of television in the critical-care area are the potential for involving the patient in stressful viewing and the need to promote unit tranquility. Allowing limited television viewing alleviates anxiety in some patients, and channels may be dedicated to the use of videotapes and closed circuit for patient teaching. Earphones or remote controls will not add to the unit sound levels.

Although necessary, signals from patient call systems, monitor alarms, and telephones add to the sensory overload in the critical-care unit. They can increase the patient's anxiety level and disturb or prevent needed sleep. These auditory alarms are a source of irritation to staff, who may turn them off in self-defense because of the tension they produce. Without reducing their importance or sense of urgency, such signals can and should be made pleasant sounding. The ICU has enough stress without the irritating alarm systems. Musical tones in varying combinations may be used and the sound intensity modulated at the lowest level that will alert the staff. These techniques, combined with appropriate patient and family instruction as to the purpose of the signals, and prompt response by the staff can result in an increased sense of confidence, efficiency, and order.

Locating individual staff members in large units can be a major difficulty.

Use of intercoms linked to all rooms or loud calling have proven disturbing and unnecessary. A system may be installed whereby the nurse activates a switch, indicating at the central station that a member of the staff is in a particular area or room. Correctly used, the system allows the charge nurse to easily locate staff. When used with the patient assignment sheet, it permits a fairly accurate location of specific individuals.

Various mechanisms can aid in the control of sound transmission. Floor coverings that absorb sound should be selected. In patient care areas the floor should be covered with a durable tile that cleans easily and requires no waxing. Traffic areas and the central station may have tile or low-pile, stain-resistant carpeting that meets state and federal codes. This will help absorb conversation, movement of equipment, alarms, ringing telephones, and transmission of sounds from room to room. In any case, portable equipment and carts should be ordered with large casters or wheels to allow easy movement of bulky, heavy equipment.

Wall construction in the critical-care area should be of materials with low sound transmission characteristics. They may be covered with a washable vinyl that is more sound absorbent than a washable enamel paint. Drapes or shades of acceptable fireproof fabric may be used as an attractive window covering and to absorb sound. They must be easy to clean, and a specified routine for cleaning should be established. Doorways may be offset to reduce transmission of sound rather than placing them in symmetrically opposed positions.

Ceilings should be covered with acoustic tile to prevent sound reverberations. If possible, avoid painting acoustic ceiling tile because this will reduce its sound-absorbing capacity.

Maintaining a comfortable thermal environment for all patients, regardless of age or level of illness, staff, and visitors is an impossible task. The emphasis should be on patient comfort, since the staff and visitors can alter their attire as needed. The inability of patients to control this aspect of their environment may serve as a source of psychological stress, increasing cardiac work. Deviations from patients' normal comfort range in temperature and humidity may physiologically increase metabolic activity and again increase cardiac work when the cardiovascular system is already stressed. Lighting and electronic equipment generate heat, which can add to the discomfort in confined spaces. Another problem is odors from cleaning agents, medications, wound or gastrointestinal drainage, elimination processes, or foods. Odors may cling to curtains and linens unless the air is exchanged frequently.

Many state codes for critical-care units include a requirement for air conditioners as a method of temperature and humidity control. The U.S. Department of Health, Education, and Welfare's *General Standards for Construction of Hospital and Medical Facilities* makes the following recommendations for intensive care and cardiac care units: the temperature range must be between 70° (21° C) and 80° F (27° C) and the relative humidity must fall between 30% and 60%.[7] A minimum of two changes of outdoor air an hour and not less than six total air changes an hour are desirable. Each patient area should have individual temperature controls. Bed positions should be carefully determined relative to window locations, door openings, and air-conditioning outlets to minimize excessive air movement around the patient.[4] Humidity levels should be maintained above 50% to minimize shock from static electricity.[8] It also provides better humidification of the patient's minute volume, which is usually increased because of the hypermetabolic state of most critical-care patients.

Natural and artificial illumination will have an impact on the patient's room. The design of the unit should use natural light to the best advantage and modify or control it as necessary to provide the desired quality of room illumination. Sunlight may be controlled by use of exterior overhangs, louvers, tinted or reflective glass, or by the use of curtains, shades, or blinds. The problem of cleaning can be solved by using thermal windows manufactured with blinds between two panes of glass.

Artificial room lighting must be able to satisfy several needs. For examination of the patient and emergency care, a light that provides a minimum of 100 shadow-free footcandles (fc) effective over the entire bed area is required.[9,10] General room lighting should be adaptable to the patient's needs. Bright ceiling lighting that reflects from shiny equipment and wall surfaces is uncomfortable and frequently intolerable to the supine patient. Noninstitutional, indirect lighting at varied levels and intensities can soften the atmosphere, allow relaxation, and provide visual variety. Local lighting for reading should produce 20 to 30 fc.[10] Since the care and observation of patients continues at night, low-level, low-intensity (2 to 4 fc) light is necessary for the nurse to safely move about the bed and room. A wall-mounted rheostat (dimmer), which will adjust to various lighting intensities, is preferred over an on/off switch.

Environmental considerations must include methods of establishing privacy for the patient. Normally, as healthy individuals, we establish our own private space (territorial right) and use various mechanisms to prevent uninvited intrusion. These mechanisms include holding people at a distance, withdrawing, merging into the anonymity of a crowd, or using physical barriers. Hospitalization reduces the alternatives available to the patient for privacy. To provide the necessary treatment and care, the hospital staff must invade the little private space that can be maintained. Discomfort, tension, and anxiety are increased when one's private space is violated by intrusive sights, smells, and sounds. If it is accepted that privacy is imperative for maintaining the individual's integrity, then providing for privacy becomes mandatory. The need for confidential communication, emotional releases, and attending to bodily functions requires privacy. Screens, blinds, or curtains establish a visual physical barrier and define the patient's private space. When feasible, permission to enter this space should be obtained from the patient. Sound intrusion may be controlled by closing doors to individual rooms and by using wall materials with low sound transmission characteristics. Doors and an adequate air exchange system help control odors. The successful critical-care unit must have built-in positive qualities that will ensure the care of the hospitalized patient with dignity and compassion. The patient must be provided with mechanisms to at least partially control the amount of contact he wishes to make with surrounding events.

Safety factors, both electrical and sanitary, must be included in environmental considerations. During recent years there has been a proliferation in the development and use of patient care instrumentation. These technological changes are affecting even the smallest hospitals. The advance in electronic patient care instrumentation has improved diagnostic and monitoring capabilities, but has resulted in a complex electrical environment that routinely exposes the patient to a variety of electrical hazards. The major hazard existing for patients in critical-care units is that of electric current passing through the body. Currents that can be felt are termed *macroshock* and register at levels greater than 1 milliampere (mA). The effects of macroshock may be tingling (1 mA), inability to let go because of contraction of the flexor muscles (16 mA), and severe pain (50 mA). At higher levels, burns and tissue damage, respiratory arrest, and ventricular fibrillation may occur.[11] Secondary injuries may occur as a result of startle reactions. Macroshock injuries are usually attributed, singly or in combination, to poor equipment design, defective or damaged equipment, improper use, and inadequate or lack of equipment ground. These problems can be effectively prevented by having all electronic instrumentation completely checked by knowledgeable biomedical engineering personnel when it arrives in the unit and at specified periodic intervals. The architect/designer should provide an adequate intact grounding system. Education programs on the proper use and maintenance of these devices should be provided by knowledgeable critical-care and biomedical engineering staff members.

The more insidious danger, however, results from microshock currents below the perception threshold (<1 mA). In normal everyday activities, these currents are common, harmless, and go unnoticed. In the critical-care unit conductive pathways (i.e., external pacemaker catheter, saline-filled central venous pressure [CVP] catheter, and/or pulmonary arterial catheter) are provided directly to the heart. Minute levels of current such as 20 microamperes (μA) will cause ventricular fibrillation, which if not detected and terminated immediately, will result in death. The causes of microshock are attributed to the same causes mentioned for macroshock. A major cause of microshock alone is an inherent normal feature of all line operated equipment, leakage current. Electronic instrumentation cannot be insulated to effectively and completely prevent the flow of electricity from its electrical components to other conductive parts such as the metal frame. The first approach to drain away the leakage current is to attach a third conductive wire (ground wire) to the metal case, add to the power distribution system a ground wire that terminates in the earth, and have the two connected by a power plug ground pin. Unfortunately, this system is subject to breakage, wear, abuse, and normal deterioration. If the grounding system does not remain continuous from the metal case of the device to the earth, an alternative conductive pathway to the ground is provided through the myocardium. These leakage current levels ($>20 \mu A$) are sufficient to present a major hazard to the patient's life (Fig. 5-6). A recent requirement for electronic instrumentation for patient application is a second system designed to protect the patient from leakage current even if the ground feature fails. This involves a new type of circuitry known as *isolated input*. Isolated input prevents the development of an electrical circuit for leakage current that would include the patient as part of the pathway.

Since leakage current can be a major hazard to the patient, preventive measures include those discussed under macroshock. In addition, the architect/designer should assure an adequately grounded electrical distribution system with each duplex output placed on a separate circuit. Outlets must have the ground connections bonded together to provide a single common ground for each patient.

The unit policy concerning electrical safety and monitoring should be established to meet or exceed the requirements of the regulating authorities (JCAH, etc.). Records, available for inspection, should be maintained by the biomedical engineering department in close cooperation with the critical-care unit committee.

Effective sanitation must be promoted as an important safety feature. The design must allow ease of cleaning while the patient is in the bed area and after transfer from the unit. Bedside supplies should be stored in closed, easily cleaned cabinets to decrease the accumulation of dust and contaminants. Wall surfaces and storage units must be able to withstand frequent washings with disinfectants without deterioration or staining. Curtains must be fire retardant, washable (or disposable), resist staining, and be changed at specified intervals.

Dirty utility rooms should be provided with a large flush sink for disposal of wound or gastric drainage, blood, secretions, vomitus, feces, and urine. The knee-operated faucet should mix hot and cold water, and have an attachment to rinse containers without splashing. A steam hopper for bedpans is also necessary. The utility room walls should be tiled to at least the 6-foot level and have waterproof electrical outlets, a floor drain to allow hosing when the flush sink overflows or when one of the above materials is dropped, splashed, or spilled, and for routine cleaning.

When many disposable items are used, trash containers can overflow quickly. The size, location, and liners of trash containers should be convenient as well as sanitary. The housekeeping department must be involved in the selection, location, and emptying schedule.

A separate container at each bedside such as an empty irrigating solution

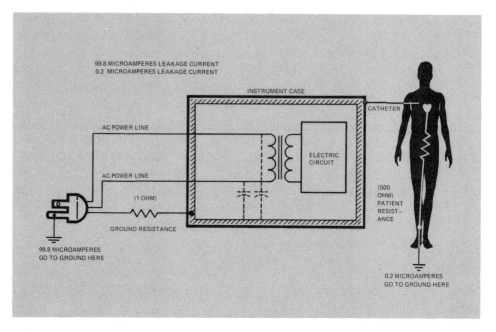

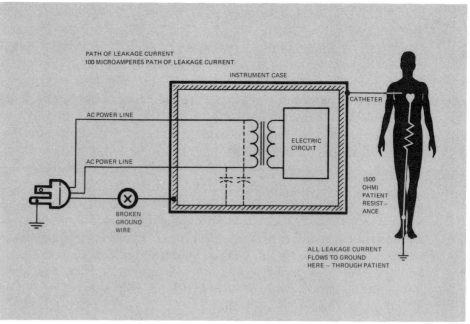

Fig. 5-6. Path of leakage current when grounding wire is defective. (From Patient Safety, 1971, Medical Electronics Division, Hewlett-Packard Co., Waltham, Mass.)

bottle with screw-on cap that can be used for disposal of needles or scalpel blades prevents inadvertent punctures. Many hospitals have specified containers for needles; they should be kept at the bedside as well as in the medication area and on the emergency drug cart. A container for used syringes should also be kept at each bedside. By providing an adequate number of disposal containers, the bedside area can remain neat and safe.

A method for dressing change and disposal of used dressings should be established and strictly enforced. To decrease the possibility of transmitting organisms, disposable equipment is desirable when possible, particularly for the isolated or infected patient. This includes washbasin, emesis basin, thermometer, bedpan, urinal, suction tubing, suction containers, ventilator tubing, etc. When a patient is critically ill and has an impaired defense system, every measure possible should be taken for protection. Methods of preventing nosocomial infection by transmission of organisms from patient to patient should be reviewed frequently. Surveillance by the nurse epidemiologist and bacteriologist can quickly identify problems. The unit policy for sanitation and infection control should be established, written, and monitored by the nurse epidemiologist, bacteriologist, housekeeper, critical-care nurse, and physician directors. In addition, a good orientation of staff in electrical safety and infection control helps the program succeed.

EQUIPMENT CHOICE

Critical-care units involve substantial electronic instrumentation. The equipment is required to function for prolonged periods of time with minimal attention and is used by hospital staff under stressful, tension-producing conditions. It is generally agreed that use of electronic monitoring devices does not reduce the number of trained staff required, but it can relieve them of some of the monotonous data-logging duties.[11] Electronic patient care instrumentation should make the care of the patient easier or improve the quality of care, but presently, it cannot remove the requirement for human interpretation and judgment.

Selection of equipment is a crucial step to be taken with much thought, review, and evaluation. A cost-effective concurrent decision may be to standardize equipment used in several hospital areas. Physicians, nurses, and technical personnel from the involved areas should be represented with the biomedical engineers and administrators in the decision-making process. The equipment should be selected in a systematic manner by the team that will be using it.

A survey of the equipment in the institution should be undertaken. Then the participants should review identified needs not being provided presently and determine if a new type or simply more of the same equipment is needed and if the manufacturer is satisfactorily providing service. A review of the literature available on the equipment being considered should be conducted.

The review of as many manufacturers as possible will provide insight into the state of the art, current trends, possible future trends, or problems. The group should identify the parameters required of the equipment presently and in a projected 10-year time frame. Nursing/medical parameters required should be reviewed by biomedical engineers and a set of electronic specifications should be developed. Evaluations of equipment, such as those conducted and published by the Emergency Care Research Institute in *Health Devices*, should be reviewed to assist in narrowing the acceptable choices.

Suitable competitive equipment that meets the requirements should be reviewed again. The group participants should then meet with the sales representatives, have the equipment shown and demonstrated, arrange for the trial use of the equipment in the unit, review service records of the companies and how rapidly it can be provided, and compare equipment warranties. It is helpful to talk to staff in other institutions who are using the equipment under

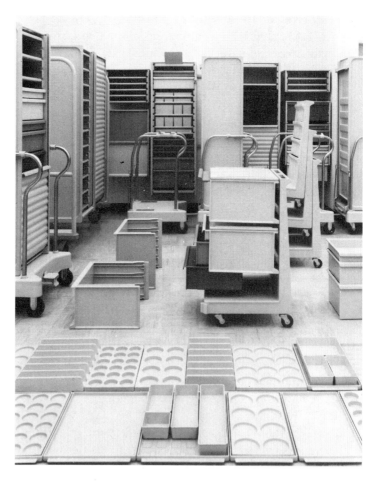

Fig. 5-7. Display of components for modular supply system. (Courtesy Herman Miller, Inc., Zeeland, Mich.)

consideration. The manufacturer can supply a list of these institutions. Revising the original parameters established may be indicated at this point, and then a final decision is made as to the equipment requirements. Acceptable manufacturers should be provided with final equipment requirements and parameters, and then requested to submit cost quotations.

Successful completion of this systematic approach to equipment selection should result in satisfaction of user requirements, improved and easier patient care, and an effective relationship with the selected manufacturer.

STOCKING AND SUPPLYING THE UNIT

Supplying the critical-care unit is usually developed in relationship to the hospital-wide system already in use. The list of equipment and supplies needed to deliver high-quality care is extensive. Recently, industrial methods of moving and storing supplies have been used effectively by health care institutions.[12] These systems vary considerably from the supply closet stocked from large movable supply carts to the modular exchange system (Fig. 5-7). Whether a cart or modular exchange system is selected, a specific area for storage must be included in the unit design.

REFERENCES

1. Kiely, W. F.: Critical care psychiatric syndromes, Heart Lung **2**(1):54-57, 1973.
2. Soloman, P., et al.: Sensory deprivation, Cambridge, Mass., 1961, Howard University Press.
3. Leiderman, P. H., Mendelson, J. H., and Wexler, D.: Sensory deprivation: clinical aspects, Arch. Intern. Med. **101**:389-395, 1958.
4. Clipson, C. W., and Wehrer, J. J.: Planning for cardiac care, Ann Arbor, Mich., 1972, The Health Administration Press.
5. Nonflammable medical gas systems, NFPA 56F, 1970, National Fire Protection Agency.
6. Standards for medical-surgical vacuum systems in hospitals, Pamphlet P-2-1, Compressed Gas Association, Inc., 1967.
7. General standards for construction of hospital and medical facilities, Public Health service, 1969, U.S. Department of Health, Education, and Welfare.
8. Buchsbaum, W. H., and Goldsmith, B.: Electrical safety in hospitals, Oradel, N.J., 1975, Medical Economics Co.
9. Hospital Electrical Facilities, Public Health Service, 1969, U.S. Department of Health, Education, and Welfare.
10. Hospital and medical facilities—lighting for patient rooms, Public Health Service, 1967, U.S. Department of Health, Education, and Welfare.
11. Hill, D. H., and Dolan, A. M.: Intensive care instrumentation, New York, 1976, Grune & Stratton, Inc.
12. Co-struc research report, Zeeland, Mich., 1971, Herman Miller, Inc.

CHAPTER 6

Supplying the unit

James A. Van Drimmelen

The method selected for supplying the critical-care unit will have a major effect on its planning and operation. Hospital-wide patient charge practices, inventory control methods, and budgeting, purchasing, and accounting procedures will also influence the unit's supply system. Three methods are generally used for bringing supplies to patient care areas: the static floor stock, par level exchange cart, and modular equipment supply systems. Sometimes one or more of these methods are used. Plans for supplying the unit should be consistent with overall hospital supply methods. It is wise to face all issues regarding the unit's supply systems early in physical and operational planning.

Planning for efficiently locating, stocking, and dispensing of supplies is an effective technique for planning spaces and the way in which they will be used. Critical questions concerning routine and emergency supplies, backup and special needs, and ways to reduce nursing involvement in supply activities will raise prime planning issues. Supply system planning should rank in priority with decisions regarding nursing policies and procedures, patient care programs, life-support systems, and major space relationships.

Critical-care units present a special problem in materials handling techniques. The hospital must meet the routine and emergency needs of the unit as simply and directly as possible without distorting its overall systems. Those responsible for critical patient care must maintain adequate levels of routine and emergency supplies. They must also meet frequent changes in patient needs and physician orders. Failure to recognize these fundamental aspects of the critical-care unit during planning can lead to distorted solutions and excessive backup systems and supplies.

Industrial methods and modular supply and work-station equipment have become dominant elements in hospital planning. Both the critical-care planning committee and the project architect or consultant should be acquainted with the various new methods and equipment available. In the selection process, an architect's or consultant's understanding and acceptance of current modular supply systems should be probed. The architect or consultant should be able to realize the implications of modular systems for the physical plan of the unit and overall hospital operations. The person selected should be able to offer constructive support during evaluation of various available supply methods and equipment. In turn, the planning team should explore major questions related to supply systems before planning sessions begin.

Supplying the critical-care unit represents one of its major operating costs. If supply systems for the critical-care unit are to be based on efficient, cost-effective procurement, stocking, and distribution methods, the unit and the hospital cannot escape taking a hard, realistic look at current practices throughout the hospital. The issues raised and decisions made regarding supplies for the unit can affect to varying degrees most existing hospital procurement and distribution channels.

The critical-care unit staff that hopes to modify existing hospital supply methods will need the full cooperation and support of all internal suppliers. The greater the courage, foresight, and objectivity with which the planning team approaches the study of supply and work flow needs, the better the unit planning will be. In turn, it will have a more constructive influence on the various departments on which it depends. The administration must decide early in planning if it wishes to move toward consistent operations in all patient care units. If the hospital has already developed good materials management practices, the planners' task will be the simpler one of achieving goals within an existing framework.

It is advised to identify early certain conditions or parameters that will affect the unit's supply systems. There are general critical-care units and variations such as medical/surgical, pediatric, neonatal, cardiovascular, coronary, burn, and trauma critical-care units. The planning team must recognize that different care units have different supply requirements.

The unit's design, whether in new, remodeled, or existing space, will influence supply methods. Such factors as plan relationships; access to the unit; nurse travel times and absence from the patient; number, arrangement and openness of patient bed areas; and the size and location of utility rooms and supply areas will all influence supply system planning. If a new plan is being designed, there will still be an ongoing interaction between floor plan and systems, which will affect solutions for both. In planning a supply system, the following factors must be considered: the budget for initial building construction and supply equipment; whether the hospital will use existing carts or is interested in new materials handling equipment and methods; the organizational and operational structures of the hospital; and the attitudes and cooperation to be expected from other departments and the administration. Experience, attitudes, and goals within the unit will also condition the planning team's approach.

Change is another factor affecting supply systems. Elements of change should be identified by the planning group. Items to be recognized as elements of change are the kind and numbers of patients, patient care and nursing programs, kind and quantity of supplies, and changes in the use of disposable supplies. Changes in materials handling methods and hours of operations of supply and service departments can affect supply quantities. A review of past experience and an attempt to identify possible future changes will lead to an understanding of the need to find flexible solutions for supply methods, space, and equipment.

A careful study of present conditions is important if meaningful improvement or change is to be achieved. It can be said that change occurs when the pain of position exceeds the pain of transition. Evaluate present hospital methods to determine if they are the best possible. Measure how much nursing time is spent on checking floor stock, writing purchase orders and requisitions, receiving and shelving supplies, disposing of waste cartons, running and fetching, borrowing from other supply centers and nursing units, making special requests for supplies and linens, checking for outdated and obsolete supplies, and telling others where to find supplies.

Review the number of sources of supply your unit deals with. Who supplies an item, and who delivers it? Follow the flow of supplies to their origin to discover multiple flows, handling, and sources. Determine average inventory levels. Are quantities adequate for a day, week, or 6 months? Check to see if the location of supplies is consistent and convenient. Search the unit for spurious, unofficial inventories. What items are directly ordered? Check to see if patient charge systems are simple and effective. Awareness of faults in present methods will prevent their carry-over into new facilities.

Once problem areas are identified, administrative understanding and support must be gained through the development of clear, concise statements of goals and good supportive data. Cost information on redundant supplies, lost charges, and wasted nursing hours is good motivation.

AVAILABLE METHODS AND EQUIPMENT

Hospitals presently use one or more of several methods to provide needed supplies in the nursing units. Static floor stock and par level exchange cart supply systems are common. Often combinations of these systems exist in one hospital, resulting in numerous supply routes, excessive handling, duplicate stocking, and hoarding at all levels. Recently, true 24-hour exchange systems using modular storage-transport dispensing equipment have come into use in many hospitals. They offer many advantages in space use, standardization, supplies handling and control, and responsiveness to user requirements. The facility-wide methods existing in the hospital and the willingness of the administration to make and support changes must be considered in planning the critical-care unit's supply system.

Static floor stock

Traditional, and still very much a part of many hospitals, is the static floor stock method. The hospital operating at this level should give itself a critical self-examination before planning new nursing facilities. This method may be appropriate for small hospitals, but larger institutions should explore more cost-effective ways of managing supplies. In the static floor stock system, supplies are held in the units in fixed shelving. Levels of linen and medical/surgical supplies are maintained in any one or a combination of several ways. Often personnel check supply cupboards daily and prepare a list of needed items (Fig. 6-1). The order is then delivered or transmitted to various central supply and processing departments where it is individually picked, loaded into carts, and delivered to the floor. Usually, nurses shelve the supplies as they are received. Linen service personnel may shelve linen or leave a cart. In addition to a daily routine delivery, the nursing department often requests one or more additional deliveries of linens and supplies. In many hospitals the system has advanced; at least some of the cupboards are restocked by stores, central supply, or laundry personnel who make daily rounds to check shelf inventories. Then they make follow-up rounds with a cart to restock drawers and shelves. Since supply needs are not determined until supply personnel have inventoried the entire unit, this method is reactive rather than predictive.

Supplies for the pharmacy, respiratory therapy, dietary, and others may also be handled in this manner. These departments often determine their own floor supply levels with minimal nursing input and then more or less automatically restock their cupboards. Such methods are usually not responsive to the needs of a critical-care unit. To compensate, the unit staff increases the amount of routine, emergency, and backup supplies held on the floor.

Direct procurement is a frequent part of static floor stock systems. The unit staff prepares orders for special items that stores or central supply do not carry or are frequently out of stock. The orders may go directly to the vendor, but are more often transmitted through the purchasing department. The supplies are then received by hospital stores and delivered to the unit, often in a bulk 6- to 12-month supply. At times, stores will procure and deliver certain items in bulk only, also forcing the unit to receive and hold large amounts of supplies. This means that the nursing staff must unbox street cartons, shelve supplies, and dispose of waste cartons. The process brings contamination to the unit and requires large amounts of floor space and expensive nursing time.

Other prime weaknesses in the static floor stock system are lack of standardization of products and methods, poor control, outages of critical items even with generally abundant supplies, inability to group and locate supplies for convenient use, excessive time spent inventorying, requisitioning, delivering, and retrieving supplies, and the growth of multiple sources and routes. Excessive amounts of supplies in the unit encourage pilfering, borrowing, and waste. Built-in casework storage is relatively inflexible. The amount, ar-

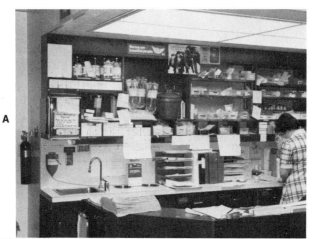

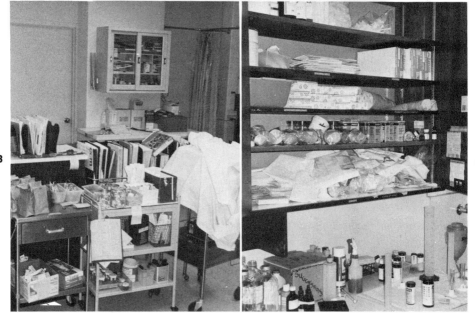

Fig. 6-1. Typical problems encountered with unplanned storage of supplies and work surface areas in critical-care areas, **B.** Note overflow of supplies onto work surfaces, **A** and **C.** Disorganization of supplies makes location and retrieval difficult. All shelves must be emptied and cleaned in place.

rangement, and location of fixed storage elements cannot be readily modified to suit changing needs.

The static floor stock system usually has separate sources, routes, and delivery personnel for nursing supplies, patient care items, pharmacy items (both prescription and nonprescription), linen, dietary, paper and office supplies, and housekeeping supplies. With this system, each supplying department has a tendency to act autonomously. Users often perceive some or all of their suppliers as unresponsive, inconsistent, and inadequate. The result is localized hoarding, direct buying, and other protective measures, which in turn creates excessive inventories, space demands, and heavy nursing involvement in supply activities. Handling patient charges, recalls, outdated and annual inventories and inspections is often complicated and time-consuming. Since each unit within the hospital tends to act more or less autonomously in relation to in-house suppliers, products and procedures are seldom effectively standardized throughout the hospital.

Strangely, although floors are often flooded with supplies, a high incidence of calls are received for missing or stat items. Under the fluctuating daily demands of each nursing unit, suppliers cannot develop good data for predicting needs. Users are not forced to analyze their needs in a systematic way so that suppliers can become more efficient and reliable. As a result, outages and delays are frequent.

Multiple locations for several different items required in a particular procedure force nurses to spend a great amount of time searching for supply items. In the static floor stock system each supplier is often given a particular cart, shelf, or niche, and supplies tend to be located according to space availability and the supplier's convenience rather than logical groupings and locations. Such methods are obviously not the best for critical-care units when retrieval time is vital. As a protective measure, the nursing staff usually increases the amount of nursing supplies held at the patient's bedside. Individual room stock systems in which each room contains virtually all the supplies required for a patient usually waste time and supplies.

In summary, the greatest weaknesses in the static floor stock system are lack of standardization and control, outages of critical items even with abundant general supplies, excessive use of floor space in the unit, inability to group and locate supplies according to use, excessive amounts of time used in daily inventorying, delivery and retrieval, uncoordinated multiple sources and flows, and inflexibility (Fig. 6-1).

If a critical-care unit must use a static floor stock program because the hospital cannot or will not change supply systems, the planning team and administration must make the most effective use of methods available while retaining options for future modifications and improvement.

The critical-care staff and planning team should develop sound lists of minimal daily routine and emergency supplies. Great care should be taken to stock reasonable amounts of needed supplies without resorting to excessive backup. It may be determined that it is more efficient to deliver supplies once, twice, or three times weekly rather than daily, but preparing a list of supplies needed daily is a strong planning discipline.

Once accurate supplies lists are developed, they should be directly related to required storage. In casework storage planning, there is a tendency to fill available walls or recesses with cabinetry rather than define the amount of storage needed in terms of supplies to be held. Another frequent error is confusing work surface needs with storage needs. There is often no direct correlation between the amount of counter space required for a task and the amount of storage that may be located under or above it. The use of drawer and shelf storage units to complete or support a work counter may prove redundant and expensive. It is better to consider open counter supports if storage under the counter is not required.

Another typical reflex is the automatic placement of storage cabinets above each work counter. Verify that the storage is needed and easily accessible before requesting it.

Since fixed casework cannot be readily modified, greater care should be taken in determining the amount and design of fixed casework provided in the unit. This can be done by measuring the amount of storage currently being used by the unit or by gathering the daily supplies actually needed and analyzing the kind (drawer or shelf), dimensions, and quantity of storage units required to hold them.

Static storage units should be designed for easy reach and visibility of contents. Rapid retrieval and ease of inventory should be considered in selecting drawers and shelves. Proper labeling and standardized arrangements should make it easy for every member of the critical-care team to locate supplies. Flexibility, cleanability, and maintenance should be considered in selecting static storage units.

Unit planners should consider the entire flow of medications, nursing supplies, and linens in planning static floor stock storage units to reduce multiple handling, redundant stocks, and excessive backup systems. A constant distinction should be made between emergency and routine supplies.

The amount of supplies held at the bedside will be influenced by the nursing program and by the physical arrangement of the unit. The method for stocking bedside storage units should be integrated with the unit's overall supply systems to reduce multiple handling and redundant stock.

Bedside storage units should be movable for emergencies. Drawers that may be interchanged between central storage units and bedside units facilitate handling groups of supplies rather than individual items.

In static systems the use of small carts equipped with needed supplies to restock decentralized supply centers is generally well established. Planning should build on and improve these existing methods.

Par level exchange cart

The par level exchange cart is probably the most common method for stocking nursing units (Fig. 6-2). It is seldom used by itself, being most often combined with one or more shelf restock programs. In the true par level cart program, nursing and suppliers predetermine the amount of supplies required for a given time period, usually 24 hours. A fully loaded cart is brought to the floor and exchanged for a partially depleted cart. The depleted cart is then returned to central service or stores for restocking to the par level and held until

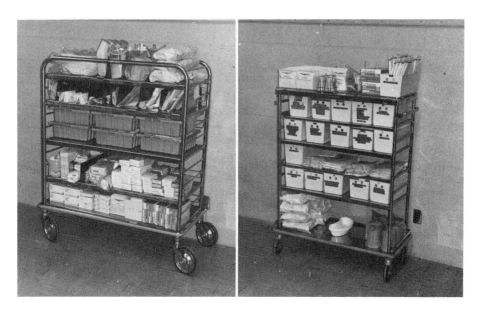

Fig. 6-2. Examples of two par level exchange carts. Carts are shrouded for transport.

the next exchange. Special supply requests are filled by a runner or pneumatic tube on a demand basis. Often, only the linen department and central stores or the central supply department will operate an exchange cart program. Other departments such as pharmacy, dietary, and respiratory therapy will be operating shelf restocking programs. Seldom does the par level exchange cart contain all the medical, surgical, patient care, and medication administration supplies required for total patient care (Fig. 6-3).

In hospitals with more advanced materials management concepts, the par level exchange cart will be loaded according to the convenience and needs of the users rather than along purely departmental lines. For instance, the pharmacy will no longer be supplying nonprescription items that could just as well be provided by stores or central supply.

When planning exchange cart supply systems the unit planners should attempt to bring daily levels of all needed supplies in one supply cart. Multiple sources and deliveries should be consolidated as much as possible.

The unit staff should prepare an accurate list of daily quotas of linen and supplies (including intravenous catheters and solutions), and then both the unit staff and its suppliers should verify the list by monitoring daily usage. Once par levels are established, the list should be finalized and used as a cart loading schedule. Periodic or continuous monitoring of daily usage will provide data for adjusting par levels.

Every effort should be made to eliminate static shelf stocking. This will reduce direct orders and bulk receiving and, consequently, the amount of supplies and static storage in the unit.

Linen levels should be adjusted to provide required amounts of linen on the exchange cart. By working together on the planning committee the unit staff and linen service can virtually eliminate all trips and calls for extra linen. Planning the linen exchange program also offers an opportunity to examine nursing and linen procedures. Bed-change packs, linen quotas and usage, and the handling of special linen needs can be reviewed at this time.

Whether the hospital has a unit dose medication program and an intravenous therapy team will have an effect on planning for medication and administration supplies. If the par level exchange cart can be stocked with intravenous therapy equipment, medications, and administration supplies, it will be more convenient for the nursing staff. These items may be transferred to medication and intravenous preparation areas.

Carts should be stationed for user convenience. This is more feasible when planning a new unit. Available space for carts is a prime consideration in planning systems for existing or remodeled space and may be the deciding factor in determining whether the system can be used. The savings to be obtained in life-cycle operating costs can make remodeling or designing to create exchange cart spaces a good investment.

If exchange carts do not exist in the hospital or unit, new ones should be purchased after criteria have been established. The following are factors to consider: volumetric efficiency and appropriateness to contents, organization of contents, ease of loading and retrieval, protection from contamination, visibility of contents, floor area required for each cubic foot of storage, mobility, and durability. If new exchange carts are being evaluated, the unit planners

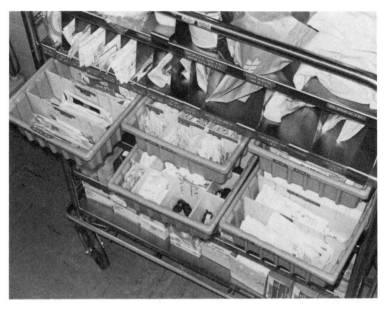

Fig. 6-3. Organization of supplies on typical exchange cart.

should consider upgrading their present system to integrated modular materials handling and work station equipment.

Modular equipment

Modular equipment supply systems are the third and newest major method for supplying the unit. They are steadily increasing in importance and use and should be given serious consideration. Modular equipment supply systems help organize supplies and can be integrated with work station equipment and furnishings. They can improve control, reduce handling, simplify or eliminate floor stock inventorying and ordering, and provide a flexible environment (Fig. 6-4, *A*). Additional benefits for the unit are simpler work procedures, the organized appearance of supplies, and improved recovery of lost charges (Fig. 6-4, *B* and *C*). Since modular supply equipment cycles through supply centers on a regular basis, centralized cleaning of the equipment becomes routine. Sanitation of modular transport dispensing equipment can be maintained at much higher levels than can sanitation of conventional fixed cabinets that are cleaned in place.

In considering whether to use modular materials handling equipment in the unit, many factors must be evaluated. Existing service systems in the hos-

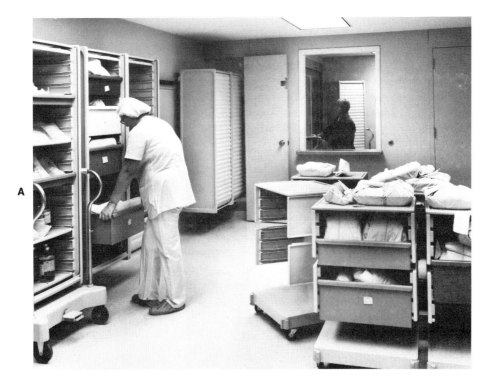

Fig. 6-4. Modular storage-transport system. **A,** Organization of supplies by use. (**A** courtesy Herman Miller, Inc., Zeeland, Mich.)

Continued.

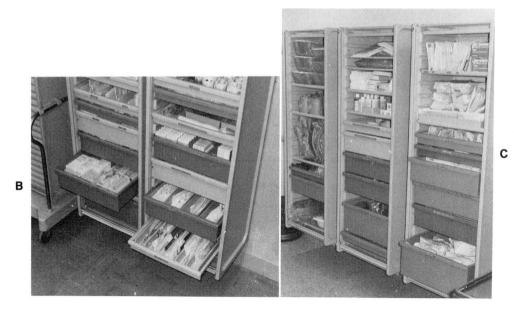

Fig. 6-4, cont'd. B, Organization by convenience of retrieval. **C,** Organization by appearance of supplies.

pital should be appraised realistically. The unit members may choose to be a pilot project for the hospital, but without at least the understanding and support of supply departments and the administration, chances for obtaining optimal results will be greatly reduced.

If the hospital has already selected a modular materials handling system the task is one of understanding and using it effectively. To gain support and clarify their thinking, those responsible for planning must clearly define and set down in writing the reasons for departing from present methods and the goals and criteria for the new system. Included should be potential benefits for patients, users, suppliers, the administration, and the hospital. Once this has been accomplished and the support of unit personnel, central supply departments, and the administration is obtained, the planning team can embark on the next step of the process.

Several points must be considered in evaluating modular materials handling equipment. The equipment falls into three general categories. Miscellaneous carts may be purchased from any of several manufacturers and are not usually part of a total system of components, even though the carts may be modular in size. Next, there are modular systems with transport units that are primarily supply carts and modular storage units that are essentially relocatable versions of casework. Finally, there are truly integrated transport, dispensing, and work station equipment systems, which are a total flexible system of modular subcontainers, drawers, shelves, storage, transport, and dispensing units. These systems offer the maximum advantage in that they fulfill virtually all the unit's transport, storage, dispensing, and work station needs.

Since the total system is modular, equipment can be constantly recombined to suit new functions without making any of its parts obsolete. Carts and storage units within the system can be assembled to suit a variety of special tasks and procedures. It is possible to create dressing carts, procedure carts, and crash carts with modular components.

Presently, there are two major manufacturers of modular materials handling and work station equipment: Herman Miller, Inc. of Zeeland, Michigan, which makes the Co/Struc system, and Monitor Products of Tacoma, Washington, which makes Unicell. The two systems have major distinctions between them, and the hospital that is evaluating the modular supplies systems should become fully acquainted with each before making a decision. Cost is not the only factor to be considered.

The type of materials used, weight and volumetric efficiency of the storage transport units, interchangeability and redundancy of parts, and rail systems supporting the storage and work-station components are to be considered. The two systems use different basic modules, one being better suited to most hospital supplies. The size of work surfaces that may be added to mobile units may be a factor, and the size and weight of modular wall-hung storage units should be considered. A transporter cart is one of the basic equipment items in both systems. The design, function, materials, and cleanability of the cart should be considered. It should be possible to both push and pull the cart and to move several carts together as in a train.

The manufacturers' experience should also be examined. A fundamental part of the modular equipment supply system is the software governing its use. Unless the unit staff has experience with the equipment, it is advised to seek guidance from professionals who have had broad experience in planning its use and installation. The hospital should seek a manufacturer who can offer competent planning, delivery, installation, and in-service and operational support.

Visits to facilities that use the systems will be helpful in making evaluations. The hospital or unit should not make a selection or begin planning with modular systems until they have visited other facilities and become thoroughly familiar with the full range of possibilities.

Modular materials handling and work station equipment will change the physical design and operations of the unit, so a decision regarding modular equipment should be made early in the planning process.

The modular system relies heavily on materials management and exchange cart concepts. Planning for a modular system is essentially the same as for par level exchange carts with some differences. Supply levels must be established, and the supplies must be assembled and packed into transport modules. This determines the organization of supplies, number of transport modules required, modular components used to assemble the transport module, and supply schedules.

Another helpful activity is the implementation of a pilot project before planning begins. The project will yield valuable data, test and adjust operational concepts, and familiarize users and suppliers with the equipment and methods proposed for the unit. Appointing a nurse coordinator to learn modular principles, develop and monitor the pilot project, and provide in-service training and operational support is important to the success of the pilot project.

Planning should include defining supply needs, systems, and storage; work centers; flow of supplies within the unit; and the selection of appropriate modular equipment. Soiled return cycles may also be handled by modular equipment systems.

At the heart of the modular system are the transporter-dispenser module, usually referred to as a *locker,* and the horizontal rail systems, which support the locker and other storage and work-surface components. Planning will include the layout of spaces and the rail systems needed; rail systems may require backing in the wall. Planning for modular systems also includes the development of specialty carts, selecting modular components, preparation of floor plans, elevations, equipment lists, and operations manuals. Early planning and coordination with the project architects is desirable.

The hospital or unit that is planning a modular materials handling system for the first time should seek the help of experienced professionals. The way in which equipment layouts are planned and supply methods are selected can affect equipment and operating costs.

The consultant or professional experienced in planning modular systems should be able to offer assistance in equipment familiarization, pilot projects, planning, documentation, start-up, and in-service use. The professional should also be able to contribute to good space planning and improved cost-effective methods.

SELECTING A SUPPLY SYSTEM

The following points can be useful in selecting a supply system:
1. How well will the system integrate with present conditions?
    a. Administratively
    b. Organizationally
    c. Operationally
    d. Physically
2. Does it fit the following criteria for software?
    a. Simple
    b. Reliable
    c. Predictable
    d. Flexible
    e. Meets special needs without distorting the system
    f. Automatically generates data on supply levels, charges, and inventory
    g. Controls supplies and charges
    h. Contains costs

      i. Involves least amount of user time

      j. Follows good infection control principles

  3. Does it fit the following criteria for hardware?

      a. Modular—interchangeable

      b. Volumetrically efficient

      c. Organizes contents

      d. Easy to load and retrieve supplies

      e. Minimum number of parts

      f. Universal, works well for any purpose in the unit or hospital

      g. Combination of carts and static components that reduces handling to a minimum

      h. Transportable and movable

      i. Sanitizable

PLANNING STEPS

Before beginning to plan it is helpful to set down existing basic conditions, broad goals, and planning steps. Following are identifiable steps in supply systems planning:

1. Select the planning team and prepare a list of tasks and a schedule.
2. Study proposed patient care and nursing and architectural space programs (if unavailable, ask pointed questions).
3. Review current hospital supply methods.
   a. Evaluate strengths, weaknesses, impact on patient care, nursing time, and hospital costs.
   b. Inventory current supply levels versus daily needs.
   c. Study supply systems paper flow.
   d. Check how many supply sources exist and who delivers.
   e. Record how much nursing time is spent in supply activities.
4. Establish criteria and objectives for the supply system.
5. Select the supply system to be used.
6. Plan the unit for supplies.
   a. Kind and amount of supplies and storage
   b. Location of supplies
   c. Stocking and/or materials handling methods
   d. Effect on floor plan
7. Document the supply system plans and evaluations; the operation manual (describes the supply system) is one type of documentation.
8. Implement the plan; stock the unit, move in, and start up.

PLANNING TEAM

The planning team should include users, suppliers, administrators, and planners. Users are represented by unit nurses and nursing administration. A single nurse is usually adequate for nursing representation, but that nurse should consult with and enlist the aid of a representative group within the nursing department. All departments providing goods and services, such as stores, central supply, pharmacy, respiratory therapy, dietary, linen, house-keeping, and any others who will actually bring supplies to the unit, should be included. The laboratory and similar departments should be consulted if they are providing even small quantities of supplies. Department representatives need not be included in all planning sessions but they should be consulted frequently. Joint meetings are useful for developing good communications and bringing to light wasteful multiple handling and duplication of services.

The adminstration should be kept informed and participate in planning, particularly in issues that may affect other departments and overall hospital operations.

PLANNING TIME

A tendency in most hospitals is to underestimate the importance of starting good supply planning before floor plans are formulated. The time period required to complete supply planning is also usually underestimated. Time schedules should take into account the normal pace with which the hospital's committees and planning groups move, the decision steps through which any planning must pass, and other duties and time pressures that fall on planning team members. A period of 1 year before plans go out to bid is not excessive for a fairly major project, particularly if supply systems serving the entire hospital must be examined. The sooner systems planning is done, the greater the opportunity to influence the architectural program and plans. Failure to plan for supplies before schematic or design development plans are completed will mean that this vital part of unit activities must be planned to fit into existing solutions.

BIBLIOGRAPHY

Coherent structures materials management system, Zeeland, Mich., 1976, Herman Miller, Inc.
Co/Struc locker packing handbook, Zeeland, Mich., 1976, Herman Miller, Inc.

Housley, C. E.: Provocative approaches to material management, Dimens. Health Serv. **51**(10): 32 38, 1974.

POLICIES AND PROCEDURES

One of the most neglected areas in a health care institution is the writing and revision of policies and procedures. It is generally considered drudgery and receives the lowest priority. However, with regulatory agencies assuming more authority in health care delivery, policies and procedures are being carefully scrutinized. It is no longer acceptable to have the policy and procedure manual continually unavailable to the unit staff because it is being revised.

Written policies and procedures as well as a method for enforcement assure to some degree maintenance of an accepted standard of care for the critically ill. If a policy or procedure is consistently disregarded, perhaps it should be reviewed with those who violate it. The final decision as to compliance remains with the nursing/medical leadership staff.

Christopher W. Bryan-Brown (Chapter 7) discusses administrative policies as regulated by the JCAH for special care units. He identifies each standard and then interprets it with examples and a rationale that can only come from many years as a "buck stops here" director.

Sharyl Justham Verillo (Chapter 8) has dissected the policies and procedures and identified specific steps to be followed in their preparation and approval. She reminds us in advance of all those miscellaneous items and lists that result in a smoother functioning unit. For example, she suggests listing telephone numbers of physicians and nurses and making them available to avoid the frantic 3 AM search in a moment of crisis.

Both Bryan-Brown and Verillo have had sufficient critical-care clinical experience to appreciate the absolute necessity of identifying and enforcing regulations and expectations as identified in the policy and procedure manuals.

CHAPTER 7

JCAH standards

Christopher W. Bryan-Brown

The Joint Commission on Accreditation of Hospitals (JCAH) recently revised the Special Care Units section of the Accreditation Manual for Hospitals. The standards became effective for accreditation decision purposes on January 1, 1979. This document recognizes the existence of separate, incoordinate special care units, but does not endorse them. The principle is stated, "Special care units, as appropriate for the hospital, shall be developed for patients requiring extraordinary care on a concentrated and continuous basis."[1] A special care unit is one that provides specialized or intensive care continuously on a 24-hour basis.

> **Standard I:** *Each special care unit shall be well organized and integrated with other units and departments of the hospital. The scope of services provided in each special care unit shall be specified.*[1]

The relationship of a special care unit to other units must be identified within the overall hospital plan. The plan shall include guidelines for transferring and referring patients requiring services that are not provided in the special care unit. Written admission and discharge criteria are required. An example is given in the following discussion on administrative policies.

ADMINISTRATIVE POLICIES
Admission policies

The policy of admitting patients to the ICU will be flexible and depend on established priorities and the number of beds available. The following categories of patients will qualify for admission to the ICU:

Direct admission
1. Multiple injuries, car accidents, industrial accidents, penetrating wounds of the abdomen or chest, and burns, depending on degree of burn and percentage of total body surface area involved

2. Severe, acute respiratory failure that cannot be cared for elsewhere
3. Shock (hemorrhagic, septic, cardiac)
4. Critically ill patients transferred from another hospital
5. Acute intoxication from poisoning
6. Patients undergoing renal dialysis

Transfer of in-hospital patients

1. Operative or postoperative catastrophe
2. High-risk preoperative and postoperative patients and those requiring specialized monitoring and care
3. Shock (hemorrhagic, septic, cardiac)
4. Critically ill patients requiring specialized diagnostic and therapeutic procedures; includes patients with pre-existing cardiorespiratory or renal disease requiring specialized techniques
5. Acute cardiac, respiratory, or renal failure
6. Other critically ill patients requiring intensive medical care

Decisions on admission of patients

All requests for admission of patients to the ICU should be directed to the resident staff of the ICU. An admission from outside the institution has to be confirmed by the attending physician of the unit.

The patient must fulfill the criteria for admissions described previously; the senior resident of the ICU will make the decision of accepting the patient for admission to the unit. Refusal of patients for admission should be reviewed by the attending staff of the ICU.

Discharge policies

Patients will be discharged from the unit when the ICU staff believes there is no further need for intensive monitoring and treatment. The ICU will not be responsible for arranging private duty nurses when patients are ready to leave. Discharge of a patient from the ICU will not depend on the availability of private duty nurses. The referring physician or the referring service will be informed of the patient's discharge as far ahead as possible.

In emergencies, patients will be transferred out of the unit without prior formal notification of the referring physician or the referring service. The hospital administration is empowered to use any hospital bed in an emergency.

The establishment of priority is a function of ICU staff members, since they have to assess the possible benefits a patient may derive from the unit against the availability of beds and needs of other patients.

Organization of the medical staff

Standard II: *Each special care unit shall be properly directed and staffed according to the nature of the special patient care needs anticipated and the scope of the services offered.*[1]

The director. The director is required to be an active member of the medical staff with recognized special training and demonstrated competence in a specialty related to care rendered in the unit. These criteria are vague because no established training program for critical-care physicians exists as yet. Several other points have been included such as the director's responsibilities for carrying out established protocols and providing overall direction, review of services, etc. Two notable responsibilities of the director are as follows:

> . . . making decisions . . . for the disposition of patients when patient load exceeds optimal operational capacity.
>
> A qualified designee shall be readily available for administrative and consultative decisions when the medical director of the special care unit is unavailable.[1]

The ICU committee. The standard also calls for an ICU committee that shall meet at least quarterly and appropriate medical staff coverage. The role of the unit staff must be defined. Following is an example of the organization of the medical staff from a multidisciplinary ICU, which operates under a department of surgery:

Regular staff
1. Director of the unit
2. Surgical attendings assigned by the chairman of the department of surgery
3. Two or three surgical residents assigned for periods of about 3 months
4. One anesthesiology resident
5. Other residents who elect or are appointed to be full-time members of the ICU staff

Specialty consultants. Specialists from departments such as cardiology, medical, respiratory therapy, infectious diseases, hematology, and renal may be consulted as needed.

Decisions on diagnosis and treatment. The referring physician or the referring service will actively participate in the patient's total care throughout his stay in the ICU.

All patients admitted to the ICU will be subject to appropriate protocols; departure from existing protocols will be permitted only in the presence of strong contraindictions and only after approval by the director of the unit.

Only residents permanently assigned to the ICU are permitted to write orders, with prior knowledge of the senior resident of the ICU. Consultant residents are not permitted to write orders.

The final decision and diagnostic workup and treatment of patients with acute metabolic, cardiac, or respiratory problems will be made by the ICU staff. Final decisions on mechanical, technical, and surgical problems remain the sole responsibility of the referring physician or the referring service.

When conflicts in the decision-making process arise regarding the diagnosis or treatment of ward service patients, the problem will be referred to the chairman of the department of surgery. When total disagreement exists between a referring physician and the staff of the ICU, the referring physician has the option of requesting a consultation with the chairman of the department of surgery or removing the patient from the ICU.

It is important to note that this procedure is sanctioned by the board of trustees of the institution. It is also an ICU that is run as a division of a surgical service.

In other institutions patients may be admitted by physicians who continue to take responsibility for the patient's general and critical care. In specialty units, the scope of the unit as well as the privileges of the users must be spelled out.

Nursing care requirements

One requirement of nursing care is proper supervision carried out by adequate numbers of qualified permanently assigned staff. The unit nurse supervisor or head nurse shall participate in committee activities concerned with the unit.

> **Standard III:** *All personnel shall be prepared for their responsibilities in the special care unit through appropriate orientation, in-service training, and continuing education programs.*[1]

This standard lists areas in which the nursing staff should be competent and dictates that all personnel have at least annual education relating to safety, infection control, and cardiopulmonary resuscitation. Opportunities are to be provided for appropriate personnel to attend outside education programs. Documentation of these activities is required.

UNIT POLICIES

> **Standard IV:** *The provision of patient care in special care units shall be guided by written policies and procedures.*[1]

Following is a minimal list of written policies necessary for providing patient care:
1. Admission and discharge
2. A procedure for notifying both patient and his family of the identity of the physician primarily responsible for his care, and a system for keeping the patient informed of changes in his condition
3. Storage, procurement, and maintenance of equipment and drug stocks
4. Infection control
5. In the event of equipment failure or breakdown
6. Safety practices
7. Traffic control, including visitors
8. Hospital disaster plan
9. Specification as to "who may perform special procedures, under what circumstances and under what degree of supervision"
10. Standing orders
11. Special emergency treatment protocols

A useful method of informing the patient and family about the special care unit is to provide a brochure with most of the details required by this standard.

"Such policies and procedures must be approved by the medical staff through its designated mechanism and shall be reviewed at least annually, revised as necessary, dated to indicate the time of the last review, and enforced."[1]

Admissions of personnel to the unit

1. Admission to the unit will be limited to those with specific purposes.
2. All persons entering the unit must identify themselves and their purpose to the receptionist or charge nurse.
3. All persons entering the unit must wash hands and properly gown before proceeding to the patient.
4. Staff members will wear uniforms provided by the institution and will be required to change into street uniforms or cover their unit uniform with a gown or lab coat when leaving the ICU.
5. No traffic will be permitted to use the unit as a thoroughfare.
6. Supporting services will supply the unit by means of a transfer cart in the corridor.

Personnel uniforms

1. Uniforms worn in the unit will be changed no less than once a shift.
2. Persons with long hair will groom it in such a manner that the possibility of contamination of wounds will be minimized.

Visitors

1. Visitors will gown before entering patient area.
2. Visitors are limited to two persons for each patient during the following hours: 9 AM to 3 PM and 4:30 PM to 9 PM.

Handling of equipment

1. All personnel will be required to scrub their hands between patient contacts.
2. Dressings will be changed by physicians and nurses as indicated and under clean conditions requiring gloves, masks, and sterile Mayo setups. The patient shall be masked when indicated.
3. All bed linen will be changed a minimum of once daily, and in those patients with staphylococcal or similar infections, once each shift.
4. Used dressings shall be double bagged for disposal. No soiled dressings are to remain in patient care areas.

Unit design and equipment

> **Standard V:** *Special care units shall be designed and equipped to facilitate the safe and effective care of patients.*[1]

This is a design standard, giving requirements for assuring both maximum patient visibility as well as privacy; floor covering, wall coloring, lighting, isolation rooms when feasible, and intercommunicational alarm systems between the patient's bedside and nurses' station are also addressed. Adjustable beds with adequate space around them for equipment use are required. Following are specific items that should be readily available for use when needed:

1. Oxygen and compressed air
2. Ventilatory equipment and airways
3. Cardiac defibrillator with synchronization capability
4. Respiratory, cardiac and, when required, intravascular pressure monitoring
5. Transvenous pacemaker
6. Sets for thoracotomy, thoracentesis, tracheostomy, and vascular cutdown
7. Infusion pumps
8. Adequate suction systems, related equipment, and electrical outlets
9. Portable x-ray machines
10. Scale for weighing bed patients
11. Emergency carts must be available and maintained

Clinical laboratory services shall be available 24 hours a day. This service shall have the capability to perform all necessary laboratory tests such as blood gas analysis, electrolyte determinations, and osmolality.

Microbiology services are to be readily available. The standard also calls for adequate arrangements for the supply of blood, hemodialysis, diagnostic radiology services, storage of biologicals, electrical safety, preventive maintenance, and infection control.

> **Standard VI:** *Specific purpose special care units may be established as determined by the patient needs of the community and only as supported by the resources available to the hospital.*[1]

CONCLUSION

The process of regulating health care delivered in special care units is as yet only partially implemented and in a state of constant change. External agencies seem influenced by three major forces: organized public opinion, a perceived need to reduce costs, and a desire to cut waste and inefficient and inadequate service. So far, the medical staff still has a major role in determining the implementation of standards. Increasing demands are made for documentation both of what should be done and what has been done. The newer regulations will be harder for some smaller institutions to implement. This may lead to the increased centralization of critical-care facilities with a future concentration on efficient patient retrieval.

REFERENCE

1. Accreditation Manual for Hospitals, Chicago, 1979, Joint Commission on Accreditation of Hospitals.

CHAPTER 8

Administrative considerations

Sharyl Justham Verillo

The terms policies and procedures are often used interchangeably, which causes confusion as to their purpose. A policy is a definite course of action adopted for the sake of expediency; a procedure is an operational method, the manner in which to proceed with the action. Both are guidelines that promote efficiency and curtail confusion. Presently, a collection of policies and procedures is required by the JCAH for hospitals in general and individual departments specifically. When the site inspection team visits a hospital, it may scrutinize the manuals containing various policies and procedures.

When compiling the manual for a new critical-care unit, copies of hospital policies, nursing department policies, and nursing department procedures are needed. Furthermore, policies and procedures specific to critical care must be formulated and added to the existing material.

A copy of hospital policies should be requested from the appropriate person in the administrative offices, and nursing department policies and procedures obtained from the nursing office. Policies and procedures must be jacketed separately to avoid confusion. Whether hospital and nursing department policies are kept under one cover depends on personal preference and the size of the institution. A three-ring binder is easy to use, and clear plastic covers for individual sheets prevent soiling and damage. Plastic covers are particularly useful for unit procedure manuals because they tend to become ragged rather quickly.

All manuals should be systematized for easy reference. For instance, a policy manual could first be divided into sections such as unit, nursing department, and hospital. These sections could have color-coded pages and/or dividers and be designated by a number or letter. Each policy should be placed in the appropriate section alphabetically and paginated with an alphabetical listing by section in the table of contents. Policies added after the pages are numbered could be designated alphabetically until the manual is redone. For instance, page 7 could be followed by added pages 7a, 7b, 7c, etc. They in turn would become 8, 9, 10, etc. when revision takes place.

All manuals should have a front sheet with the signatures of the hospital administrator, director of nursing, and medical director of the unit. Documents specific to the unit should also have the signature of the nursing coordinator on the front sheet.

All policies and procedures should be reviewed annually. Changes relating specifically to the critical-care unit should be approved by departmental committees, and documentation of changes placed in the committee minutes. All changes should be dated and signed.

It is imperative to have two complete sets of policy and procedure manuals. One should be available to the staff at all times and should therefore be kept in the unit. The second set should be kept in the coordinator/supervisor's office as a backup. In addition, the original and a few copies of each policy and procedure should be filed to be available as replacements and when requested by other ICUs.

A committee for the express purpose of developing policies and procedures for the critical-care unit should be formed prior to the opening of the unit. This committee should consist of, but not be limited to, representatives from the administrative, nursing, and medical departments. The committee should be charged with the responsibility of developing administrative and clinical guidelines as well as defining the philosophy and objectives of the unit. The more closely the committee members are associated with the unit the more successful the work will be. Operationally, it is usually better to have one team working on policy statements and a second group developing procedures. The time necessary to accomplish these goals will depend on the motivation, experience, and cohesiveness of the committee. However, weekly meetings beginning 2 months prior to the opening are not excessive for the job to be done. All policies and procedures should be written according to requirements of local, state, and federal regulatory agencies.

Policy and procedure review should be on the agenda of all critical-care committee meetings, since changes and additions will be ongoing between annual revisions. Proper maintenance of policy and procedure manuals is time-consuming and requires attention to detail. It is inefficient and defeats the designed purpose to delay review, changes, and additions of the manual until a JCAH audit is imminent. The updating should be done regularly and honestly and treated as a valuable tool.

In Standard IV, the JCAH requires each special care unit to have specific written policies and procedures that supplement the basic hospital policies and procedures.[1] This Standard is interpreted to include the following policies and procedures:

Functions and authority of the
unit director

Admission and discharge
criteria

Special procedures,
equipment, and supplies

Maintenance programs

Respiratory care

Infection control

Laboratory considerations

Standing orders

Visitors

Traffic control

Nursing leadership

Audit requirements

Uniform regulations

Electrical safety

Staff orientation

Staff continuing education

Fire, safety, and evacuation

Isolation of infectious diseases

Review of antibiotic use

Mortality and morbidity
conferences

Collection of statistical data

Nursing practice

Basic life-support programs and
certification

Advanced life-support
programs and certification

Flowers, plants, and food

Patients' personal belongings

POLICIES

Policies can be compared to rules; they are official statements of what can and cannot be done and under what circumstances. Once the purpose of the unit is defined (cardiac care, trauma, pediatrics, etc.) and the philosophy and objectives are formulated, then policies can be written.

The hospital admission policy will state classifications of patients who may not be admitted to the facility such as those with mental disorders if there is no mental health service. Similarly, a coronary care unit may exclude from admission all patients who do not have a cardiac problem as their primary diagnosis. If such details are not made a matter of policy, it is inevitable that at some time an attempt will be made to admit a patient with gastrointestinal tract bleeding. Such a situation creates the potential for all kinds of unpleasantness and administrative conflicts. Policies can be changed much easier than habits. Try to start with the ideal as envisioned by the committee, then revise the policies to keep pace with reality.

The importance of clearly defined rules for discharge cannot be overemphasized. A critical-care unit that is properly used will have a constant flow of patients. Unless a policy precludes it, there will be a tendency to keep patients in the unit longer than necessary.

The following example may clarify the importance of written policies:

Your unit has just received two intravenous infusion pumps. They were purchased after a period of testing in the unit, since the unit has a policy that states: ". . . all equipment must be used on a trial basis before purchase. Written evaluation by six employees in the category that would have use of such equipment. . . ." You know they work, since you were one of the six employees writing an evaluation. You also know that they are delicate. The evening supervisor has just come into the unit to borrow one of the infusors for another area. Without a policy it would be difficult to prevent your new delicate machine from being loaned, but in the policy manual under "E" is a statement that says, "... under no circumstance is any piece of unit equipment to leave the department without the express permission of the nursing director for critical care. ..." Saved by the policy!

Policies dealing with interdepartmental situations may be necessary, such as a priority system for patients undergoing procedures in the x-ray department, nuclear medicine, and laboratories. It may even be necessary to write a policy outlining what personal possessions patients may have with them in the unit. This policy can then be reproduced as a pamphlet to the families. It will save a lot of explanations and reduce the frantic search for lost personal articles.

Each unit is unique and will have a few special requirements, but similarities are more common. A lot of work can be saved by reviewing the policy manuals from other units as a first step. Make a list of policies required for your unit and divide the list among the committee members for actual writing. Review and revise them in the committee meetings. Circulate them to staff members one at a time. A proven method is to have the head nurse or charge nurse briefly discuss the new or revised policy at each shift report for 2 days. The policy should be placed in the communication book and initialed by the staff as it is read. The same can be done for procedures. To present the staff with bulky manuals and expect them to be read is ignoring human nature.

PROCEDURES

Just as a policy tells what can be done, a procedure details the manner in which it is to be done. In the situation of a critical-care unit the policy might state that "... hyperalimentation may be carried out when indicated by the condition of the patient and ordered by a qualified physician. All patients receiving hyperalimentation must be in a critical-care unit, recovery room, progressive unit, or a general unit with a nursing staff qualified by special instruction to manage patients receiving such treatment. ..." An example of the procedure for hyperalimentation follows:

1. Shave chest above nipple line, including sternal notch, neck, and shoulder.
   NOTE: Same as for surgical procedure.
2. Clean skin with acetone followed by a povidone-iodine (Betadine) skin preparation.
   NOTE: Do not use Betadine on patients who are allergic to iodine or seafood.
3. Place patient in Trendelenburg's position.
   NOTE: To facilitate venous distention.
4. Put on sterile gown, gloves, and mask. Place sterile drapes around area of catheter insertion.
   NOTE: Catheter placement must be considered an operative procedure.
5. Inject or apply topical anesthetic and proceed with catheter insertion.
   NOTE: Pain control is needed, since a large-gauge needle is used.

6. Instruct patient to do a Valsalva maneuver at time of needle puncture.
7. After successful catheter placement, the needle is secured, and the catheter may be sutured to the skin. Paint skin with tincture of benzoin.
   NOTE: Chest x-ray film is necessary to determine correct catheter placement and rule out injury.
8. Apply Betadine ointment to needle hub and insertion site; cover with 2- by 2-inch dressing and seal with nonporous tape.
   NOTE: Infection control.
9. After confirming proper catheter placement, adjust rate of pump.
   NOTE: Rate to be determined by physician. Do not increase rate as a means of "catching up."

Documentation. On nurses' notes or hyperalimentation form the following should be documented:

1. Date and time procedure was performed and physician's name
2. Vital signs and weight
3. Blood drawn; urine sent to laboratory for analysis, culture, and sensitivity
4. Area prepared, solutions used, sterile drapes applied
5. Topical anesthetic used
6. Length and gauge of radiopaque catheter used
7. Method of anchoring needle and catheter
8. Betadine ointment applied to hub of needle and insertion site, and sterile dressing applied
9. Chest x-ray film obtained
10. Hyperalimentation solution used, time and rate infusion begun
11. Patient's response to procedure
12. First name initial, last name, and title

Vouchers. Transactions with the following departments must be accompanied by vouchers:

1. Pharmacy—solution
2. Laboratory
3. Central supply

Caution. The hyperalimentation line must not be used for the following:

1. Central venous pressure
2. Blood transfusion
3. Piggyback of other medications
4. Intravenous push medications
5. Removal of blood for analysis

A well-written procedure tells why the procedure is being done, gives information on expected results, lists the equipment necessary, and gives an easily followed sequential outline of the actual procedure. The procedure must state whether the particular situation is covered by the consent given in the condition of admission. If not, a special consent for that procedure must be signed by the patient and appropriately witnessed. Each procedure that requires a special consent should have a copy of that consent attached to it in the procedure manual. Key points, or an explanation of precautions to be taken, should be listed briefly at a particular step in the procedure where appropriate.

The documentation format as well as any special forms required should be listed in the procedure manual with a copy of the forms attached (pp. 101 and 103). The procedure must be specific as to the category of nursing personnel allowed to perform it. If nursing personnel may not perform a particular procedure, a statement must be made as to which category of personnel may, and the nurses' role in assisting that person in carrying out the procedure must be defined.

When writing a procedure, it is helpful to list the ancillary departments that will be needed, such as the x-ray department or laboratory, so that they may be notified prior to the beginning of the procedure.

The importance of writing procedures cannot be overemphasized. Every procedure that is carried out in a special care unit must be documented in an explicit manner. The written procedure is a guide for the new employee, a reference for senior employees, and a legal document. Retain the original procedure and all revisions, carefully noting the period of time each was in effect. So long as the critical-care practitioner acts according to the guidelines set down in properly executed manuals, the hospital bears legal liability. When a patient is subjected to a procedure that is not done according to the official written procedure, the person carrying out that procedure does so without the legal protection of the institution.

RESOURCES

In addition to the formal policies and procedures, numerous types of information should be readily available in writing. The on-call schedule for physician coverage should not only be posted, but a clean copy inserted in a binder or file and kept for 1 year. The following telephone numbers, including emergency and after-hours numbers, should be kept in the unit: physicians' exchange, office, and home; all unit personnel; other appropriate hospital employees; outside agencies; laboratories; pharmacies; fire department; police department; Red Cross; poison centers; other hospitals; vending representatives; and equipment repair services.

A list of hospital employees who speak foreign languages should include not only the name and language, but the assigned unit, shift, and home phone number of the employee. The home phone number is particularly important for those who speak a more uncommon language. This information should be obtained by the personnel department when hiring staff and distributed regularly.

Since abbreviations differ from institution to institution in geographical areas, it is advisable to have acceptable abbreviations and their meanings for your particular institution approved by the medical records committee and listed in the procedure manual.

Electrical equipment should be labeled with the location of the operation manual and preventive maintenance records. It is a good idea to make copies of operating and repair instructions for new equipment in case the originals are inadvertently misplaced.

STANDARDIZED PROCEDURES

With the great advances in critical care, many responsibilities have been placed on nurses that in the past were the domain of the physician. In an effort to provide legal protection for the nurse, some states, such as California, have begun to enact legislation that expands the traditional role of the nurse. For example, the Nurse Practice Act in California divides nursing practice into four general categories: the role of the nurse as it has been recognized in the past, the nurse carrying out the orders of a physician, the nurse functioning in an emergency situation, and the concept known as *standardized procedures.* This term has been applied to procedures and protocols developed by a hospital committee of representatives from the nursing staff, medical staff, and administration.

The standardized procedure documents evidence of the nurse's education and proven competence to perform a specified procedure and provides a

---

COMMITTEE FOR STANDARDIZED PROCEDURES

Date _____

Request has been made for approval of the following procedure: _____

_____

Category of employee to be taught: _____

_____

For the purpose of: _____

_____

Instructors: _____

Qualifications: _____

_____

Course outline attached: Yes ____ No ____

Performance evaluation:

Recertification: Yes ____ No ____   Approval: Yes ____ No ____

Valid for: _____   _____
       (1 yr, 6 mo, etc.)   (Committee chairperson)

guideline for the future expansion of the nurse's role. It should in no way be considered a license to practice medicine. When writing standardized procedures for an institution, consideration should first be given to procedures that overlap into medical practice and have become common practice in the area.

Standardized procedure committee

To implement standardized procedures, an institution must form a committee of representatives from the nursing, medical, and administrative departments. The first responsibility of the newly organized standardized procedures committee is to resolve the questions of what procedures to consider, the purpose of each procedure, and under what conditions the procedure may be performed.

When standardizing procedures, a list should be made of those which have historically been the responsibility of the physician. In some hospitals this may include injection of intravenous medications, central venous pressure (CVP) monitoring, or insertion of nasogastric tubes. In other institutions these procedures may have been the responsibility of nurses for many years and have become common nursing practice; therefore, standardized procedures would be used for more advanced procedures such as arterial punctures, placement of arterial lines, and intubation. It is not the level of sophistication of the procedure that determines whether standardization is necessary, but rather who has traditionally carried out the procedure.

The committee must define the purpose of each procedure to be standardized and under what conditions the procedure may be performed. State and local requirements as well as JCAH standards must be followed at all times. Criteria for the standardized procedure must be set, defining the specific educational and clinical experience required of those who are to carry out the procedure. The extent of the education must be determined as well as provision for clinical experience.

Choosing an instructor for standardized procedures

The instructor for standardized procedures must be qualified by education, experience, and expertise. It will be the responsibility of the committee to evaluate credentials of potential instructors with these qualifications in mind. In some instances it may be necessary to request instructors from outside the institution to initiate the standardized procedures program. In small or rural hospitals, it may be advisable to send nurses to another facility for specific training to perform standardized procedures.

The competence of the nurse must be determined after formalized instruction. This may be done by written and/or oral examination as well as return demonstration in a supervised clinical experience. The committee may either determine competency by virtue of examination scores, quality of the return demonstration, or they may take the recommendation of the person who supervised the clinical experience. Reevaluation should be done at least an-

COMMITTEE FOR STANDARDIZED PROCEDURES
INSTRUCTOR APPROVAL

Date _____

_____ is approved to serve as an instructor for:
(Name)

_____

Valid for: _____   _____
(1 yr, 6 mo, etc.)   (Committee chairperson)

COMMITTEE FOR STANDARDIZED PROCEDURES
INSTRUCTOR'S REPORT TO COMMITTEE

Date _____

_____ has received instruction in _____
(Name)

_____

Hours of instruction: _____ Date(s) given: _____
Performance evaluation:

_____
(Instructor)

Qualification approved: _____ Qualification valid for: _____
(Date)   (1 yr, 6 mo, etc.)

_____
(Committee chairperson)

nually, and in some situations 6 months is advisable. Competency may be re-evaluated by scheduling updated refresher courses and re-examinations. Clinical evaluation should be continuous. Attendance at clinical and classroom sessions should be recorded on a sign-in sheet, which is dated, timed, and signed by the instructor. A synopsis of the class as well as the purpose for which the class was given should be listed on the sign-in sheet. The written examination, evaluation of the oral examination, and a document stating the nurse to be qualified to perform a specified procedure should be retained in the personnel file.

Procedures that are considered related to critical care include cardiopulmonary resuscitation and advanced cardiac life support with airway adjuncts, dysrhythmia interpretation, defibrillation, and definitive drug therapy.

NURSING PRACTICES

Nursing personnel assigned to critical-care units must have completed a course or series of classes in the care of critically ill patients. This education should be ongoing and specific to critical care. Only registered nurses who have demonstrated expertise should have the responsibility for patient care. Nursing personnel from other categories may be used as long as they are qualified by education and experience. Personnel of comparable expertise should be available to cover vacations, leaves of absence, days off, meals, and coffee breaks. In some states, the actual number of nurses necessary to care for a patient assignment is determined by law. Educational preparation for critical care should include courses in recognition and documentation of signs and symptoms of critical illnesses, including the physiological, psychological, and social needs of the patient and the family. The critical-care nurse must be able to make initial and ongoing physical assessments as well as write nursing histories and nursing care plans. A knowledge of acid-base balance and interpretation of blood gas analysis are essential and should be part of the educational program. Cardiopulmonary resuscitation, defibrillation, and dysrhythmia interpretation are skills that should range from basic to sophisticated as the nurse gains experience. Each nurse should be taught to operate and troubleshoot ventilators used in the unit. Even though many hospitals employ respiratory therapists for this function, the nurse is the only person consistently with the patient.

It is essential that nurses hired for critical care have a basic medical/surgical background and competency in administering tracheostomy care.

Practice in the safe and effective use of electric and electronic equipment should be provided. A hospital program for infection control is essential not only for nursing personnel but all ancillary departments, including housekeeping.

The institution should clearly state what areas of nursing practice are acceptable in conjunction with local, state, and JCAH guidelines. A policy must clearly delineate the nurse's responsibility for parenteral administration of fluids, including blood, blood products, electrolytes, and medications, as well as for establishing arterial line and CVP monitoring.

The nurse should be knowledgeable in the interpretation of laboratory results and capable of performing special dressing techniques when appropriate. Psychosocial skills, such as interviewing techniques and the ability to recognize and handle stress, are essential when working in a critical-care area.

All medical and paramedical personnel should be aware of the legal aspects of health care and be familiar with federal, state, and local regulations affecting their particular discipline.

Nursing practice committee

A nursing practice committee, which provides input for staffing determinations and educational programs, is advisable. This committee can address itself to the problem of reassigning unit personnel and floating outside personnel into the critical-care units. The committee may serve as an arena for the discussion of patient conditions and treatment, or lack of treatment, with provision for immediate investigation and protective measures. It may also uphold the authority of the coordinator or charge nurse in altering visiting privileges, according to the patient's condition and activities in the unit.

The nursing practice committee may wish to address itself to the subject of private duty nurses as well as emergency procedures that may be performed by the nursing staff. Committee members may monitor the presence of educational and reference materials specific to critical care in the form of journals, textbooks, and tapes.

Nursing practice policies for a surgical-respiratory intensive care unit

Registered nurses assigned to the Surgical-Respiratory Intensive Care Unit are permitted, after completion of course and in-hospital certification, to perform the following procedures:

1. Administer intravenous fluids, including initial peripheral catheter or needle insertion. Not more than 2 ml lidocaine 0.5% plain may be given subcutaneously or intradermally as local anesthetic.
2. Draw arterial or venous blood samples.
3. Administer intravenous medications, including direct administration into the vein.
4. Administer medications (narcotics and relaxants) on a sliding scale.
5. Administer blood and blood products, including blood under pressure. The nurse must remain in attendance until the administration of blood under pressure is completed.
6. Initiate and carry out cardiopulmonary resuscitation and defibrillation.
7. Attach patients' pacing wires to pacing generator and set rate.
8. Administer intravenous lidocaine at onset of critical dysrhythmias, according to accepted protocol.
9. Administer ventilation therapy and adjust controls to achieve adequate ventilation.
10. Perform nasotracheal and bronchial suction.
11. Introduce a nasopharyngeal tube to maintain an adequate airway.
12. Insert nasogastric tube.
13. Insert urinary catheters into male patients.
14. Take 12-lead electrocardiogram.
15. Charge nurse may take verbal orders in an emergency situation.
16. Remove peripheral, central venous, and percutaneous arterial lines.
17. Apply restraints for patient safety without a physician's order.

18. Change tracheostomy tubes over introducer in an emergency or for routine changes at least 72 hours after tracheostomy.
19. Apply heating pads to area with phlebitis or edema due to intravenous therapy.
20. Remove sutures when tracheostomy tube is sutured to skin and from healed cutdown sites.

Increased health surveillance is one measure the nursing practice committee can institute to protect the health of unit personnel. In addition to preventive care, required consideration may be given to health problems frequently encountered in high-risk areas. For example, Australian antigen levels must be tested frequently in areas where hemodialysis takes place. A policy should be established for follow-up of positive findings.

INFECTION CONTROL

The decision to admit or retain critically ill patients with a communicable disease or an infectious process should be made by the critical-care committee in association with the infection control committee and hospital administration. A specific area should be designated for isolation. The category of isolation should depend on the physical layout of the unit. Physical unit designs may vary from open multibed units to glass-enclosed cubicles, or a combination of both.

The critically ill patient's natural resistance will be lowered by his debilitated state, and natural barriers are compromised by insertion of lines, catheters, and tubes. Patients may have wounds from surgery, including ruptured viscera, trauma, or burns, which will require meticulous technique and careful observations. When irrigations and dressing changes are being carried out, it is advisable to close the unit to traffic whenever possible; traffic flow should be kept to a minimum at all times.

The critical-care committee must work closely with the infection control committee to establish policies, review data on infections, and review and revise policies as necessary. In determining a policy, the committee must consider federal, state, and local regulations and review infection control policies of departments that will be involved with the unit. Policy should determine if patients with infections or communicable diseases are to be admitted or retained in the unit. If certain diseases or infections are excluded, an alternate plan of care must be defined.

Hospital personnel uniform regulations as well as requirements for visitors' use of cover gowns must be stated. Explicit requirements for cleaning nondisposable equipment as well as solutions and their concentrations must be stated. Even if not required by law, every critical-care area should have a clean utility room and a dirty utility room. Personnel must strictly adhere to the distinction between clean and dirty. Disposable equipment should be used as much as possible. Housekeeping personnel should set up and maintain a schedule for cleaning the unit on a regular basis, including ceilings, walls, light fixtures, vents, all furnishings, and floors. Equipment that can be steam-cleaned should be taken to the machinery designed for this purpose. Tile floors should be flooded and vacuumed dry. Although many units now have carpeting on the floors, primarily because it is quiet, it poses many housekeeping problems because spills are difficult to remove, and odors tend to linger. The policy for housekeeping should define the responsibility of nursing, housekeeping, and maintenance personnel in this program as well as the method and solutions to be used. Policies concerning refrigerator upkeep should include cleaning and temperature checks. Separate refrigerators should be maintained for patient food and medication. Personnel should not use unit refrigerators for their personal food. Blood and blood products should be stored only in refrigeration units designed for that purpose.

Surveillance should be maintained to prevent visitors, or unit and ancillary personnel who may have infections of the respiratory tract, gastrointestinal tract, or skin, from entering the unit. Teaching aids in the form of brochures can inform visitors of conditions that preclude their presence in the ICU. A regular program should be set up for culturing patients' equipment and the environment.

It must be defined whether the infection control program is under the auspices of the epidemiologist (nurse or physician) and the cost charged to the hospital or whether a physician order is necessary. An infection control program directed by the epidemiologist is recommended. Cultures should be obtained with consideration for laboratory hours. Responsibility for obtaining cultures and sending reports must be clearly defined.

The unit coordinator must work closely with the epidemiologist or infection control nurse so that potential problems and trends are identified early. Policies will be required concerning thermometers, intravenous therapy, intravenous tubing changes, maintaining a closed urinary catheter system, as well as catheter care and the care of respiratory equipment. Terminal cleansing, sterilization, and subsequent culturing of the equipment must be the responsibility of a specific department.

LEGAL IMPLICATIONS

Because of the nature of critical care, nurses who choose to practice in this area are perhaps at higher risk for involvement in litigation. Although most hospitals include personnel in their malpractice coverage, it is advisable for every critical-care nurse to carry an individual malpractice policy. The hospital attorney and insurance carrier should review all policies and protocols. Manuals prepared by the JCAH and regulations written by the state department of public health must be available and reviewed carefully.

Nursing personnel must have specialized training and proven competency before assignment to critical-care areas. All licensed personnel must hold a valid license for the state in which they practice. Consideration must also be given to continuing education units in states that require them for relicensure.

A record must be kept of all license expiration dates; a license renewal must be presented on or before the date of expiration. Most states issue lists of names and license numbers of persons who have licenses revoked or suspended; these lists should be reviewed, especially in the case of new personnel.

Patient consent must be obtained when required, filled out properly, and witnessed. The date and time of the patient's signature should be included. If the consent is signed by a person other than the patient, that person must be legally qualified to do so. Operative consents must not contain abbreviations and must state the full procedure to be done. It must also be specific as to right, left, or bilateral.

Should the patient not speak English or the language of the country, it would be prudent to have the consent translated and signed by the person who does the translation. A list of persons who speak foreign languages should be available for instances such as this.

Informed consent must be considered in those areas and circumstances in which this consent is required. Prior to surgery it must be signed by the patient or his legal representative and the physician.

Consideration must be given to the legal requirements for treating minors in the absence of their parents and provisions of the law for treating and protecting suspected or obvious victims of child abuse.

All documentation must be clear, concise, factual, timely, and legible. All entries must be timed, dated, and signed with the first initial, last name, and title.

REFERENCE

1. Accreditation Manual for Hospitals, Chicago, 1979, The Joint Commission on Accreditation of Hospitals.

DEVELOPMENT OF NURSING PERSONNEL

To overlook the interdependence of nurse recruitment, in-service and continuing education programs, staffing, delivery of patient care, nursing salaries, benefits, and nurse/physician relationships will weaken efforts to develop a responsive and accountable critical-care team. In Chapter 9, Jane M. Kahn discusses budgeting from the point of view of the nursing leader who is responsible for the critical-care areas. She has provided a step-by-step approach to developing a fiscal program. The initial budget for a critical-care unit that is not replacing an existing facility is best described as a series of educated guesses. The occupancy rate of the unit as well as supply usage is difficult to predict in advance. Consequently, a monthly review of budgetary factors may be necessary. When operating a new unit, it is helpful to discuss in detail anticipated supply needs with the persons in charge of stores, central supply, and pharmacy. It is not unusual for a new unit to start slowly. As physicians become more certain of the value of the unit in patient care, the occupancy rate may skyrocket. A comparison of budgets from a successful unit will reveal a dramatic yearly increase.

Allocation of funds for salaries and benefits can be made based on a 1:2 nurse/patient ratio and a high occupancy figure. The real challenge is to locate and successfully recruit adequately prepared critical-care nurses, since the supply of such nurses is not sufficient to staff the increased number of critical-care beds. Ideally, nurses should be hired with critical-care experience. However, if nurses with critical-care experience are not available, nurses with a medical/surgical background can be taught the principles and practice of critical-care nursing. Although some critical-care units hire personnel without experience, it is a difficult, expensive, and time-consuming endeavor. The preparation of a critical-care nurse should include work experience in a general medical, surgical, or pediatric unit, advancing to the intensive nursing area within the unit. The next logical progression would be to a critical-care unit and finally to the critical-care service.

Among the methods of nurse recruitment are newspaper and journal advertisements. A newspaper advertisement should be specific as to the general location of the hospital, type of unit, hours to be worked, and benefits available. Publication of salaries will depend on local practice. An advertisement that does not give geographical location will fail, since commuting is one of the main determinants in a nurse's decision to accept or reject a position. Information concerning availability of nurses in various geographical areas can be requested from the National League for Nursing, 10 Columbus Circle, New York City. Such information can be used to determine where advertising money can best be spent. Libraries and the local newspaper office can provide a book listing every newspaper published in the United States and their circulation and frequency of distribution. These sources of information will allow placement of advertisements in areas most likely to yield results.

Kahn (Chapter 9) has detailed the types of information to be gathered to determine the staffing patterns required. She discusses hiring methods and staff evaluations and retention and suggests methods that may be helpful in determining the applicant's compatibility and suitability. Although present trends in hiring emphasize the use of objective techniques and tools, the intuitive response of an experienced interviewer to an applicant should not be underestimated. There is no substitute for a talk, a cup of coffee, and a tour of the facility. The applicant cannot be properly evaluated unless care is taken to promote an atmosphere conducive to relaxation. Interesting and useful information can be gathered in a seemingly casual conversation. By the same token, it is unrealistic to expect an applicant to accept a position without proper information.

A prudent hiring practice is to advise applicants of the realities of a rotation schedule and weekend and holiday coverage so that their decision is based on facts. This may prevent unpleasant situations from arising in the future. It is also important to inform applicants of the various benefit programs available to them as employees.

Each prospective candidate should be interviewed and evaluated for nursing capability and adaptability. Decisions should be based on the applicant's experience and prior evaluations. The applicant can be taken into the ICU and introduced to a patient. By also asking for a written nursing history, assessment, and plan for nursing care, many strengths and weaknesses will be identified, including the nurse's behavior under stress. This process should take 45 minutes and may be the determining factor for both parties. It may be beneficial for the applicant to be assigned to an area within the institution to provide divergent experiences prior to assignment in the new critical-care area.

With less and less clinical emphasis in basic nursing education programs, it has become necessary for health care agencies to provide both education and clinical experience for the nursing staff. In addition to the deficiencies present on entering nursing employment, rapidly advancing technology makes continuing education necessary.

Many solutions to this dilemma of practitioner preparation have been proposed, and several have been tried with varying degrees of success. A 1-year internship similar to the program used by medical schools has been discussed and implemented, but failed to gain national acceptance. A 1-year postlicensure program was funded for a brief time by the federal government. The benefits of such programs varied according to the administering institution and the caliber of participating nurses.

Presently, most newly graduated registered nurses are left to learn through their work experiences, and self-discipline. Usually the entry level nurse is literally thrown in to sink or swim. It is a credit to each of these nurses that growth and learning occur under such stressful conditions.

For the nurse who wishes to practice critical care, educational opportunities are more structured. Provided there is requisite knowledge and adequate clinical experience, the additional skills and knowledge necessary for a nurse to practice critical care can be acquired. Most hospitals, many commercial organizations and colleges and universities, as well as nursing organizations, offer programs in various aspects of critical-care nursing.

In Chapter 10, Kathryn M. Lewis has provided a candid and graphic account of the problems and justifications involved in implementing the educational program for a critical-care service. However, she goes beyond summarizing problems and identifies a variety of solutions that have proven successful in her experience. Recognizing the expense involved, she discusses a method whereby a group of hospitals can pool their resources for educational programs. Examples of lesson plans, evaluation forms, and in-service schedules are provided.

Members of the critical-care team seek innovative and challenging work and educational experiences. We have barely seen the tip of the iceberg that is the field of critical care. This section deals primarily with nurses, since it has been written by nurses who constitute the majority of critical-care workers. But think of the possibilities and impact on critical-care education when physicians and nurses will require certification in critical care, when nonregistered nurses will give a greater portion of bedside care, and when allied health personnel will share greater responsibility in critical-care units. In some hospitals as many as 30% of the patients are classified as requiring critical care. This dramatic increase is attributed in part to the advances in equipment and techniques and most likely will only increase. As the patient load increases so will the need for care-givers. All of these health workers will require educational programs designed specifically for their job category. The cost of such programs in terms of human and financial resources is tremendous. Organization and planning will be the key to success.

To build a strong and cohesive team takes time, effort, and skill. The time to start is the day final approval is granted for the construction of the unit. At that point you know the purpose of the unit and the size. A preliminary Table of Organization (TO) should be drawn to identify the level and numbers of personnel required. Recruitment from within the institution as well as from without should be initiated. Nurses hired specifically for the unit should begin a formal orientation program as soon as possible. Those nurses hired far in advance of the opening of the unit will benefit from the opportunity to work in other areas, particularly those having a close relationship with the unit. Key leadership staff, both nurses and physicians, should be appointed as early in the planning stage as possible and immediately become members of the planning team.

As soon as sufficient members of the ICU staff are identified, various mechanisms should be instituted to bring them together. As they get to know one another and have an opportunity to identify with the ICU project, the team spirit will develop. Involve everyone—physicians, nurses, clerks, aides, therapists, and ancillary personnel—at every opportunity. And do not overlook the value of social gatherings in the forging of a team!

Depending on the size and intricacy of the unit, the nurse who will be in charge of the unit will require several weeks for the final stocking and checking of the unit. This is a time-consuming project, which can be best accomplished by the nursing staff who will be caring for patients in the area. All equipment, from electrical beds to monitors, must be received, positioned, and tested. If the institution has chosen an industrial-type stocking system such as those described in Chapter 6, all the supply decisions will have been made far in advance. At this time the actual modules can be placed. If a par level exchange cart stock system is to be used, supplies will have to be unpacked, counted, and shelved. Details concerning light bulbs, flashlights, telephone books, and other minutiae must be worked out. As the opening date draws closer, more and more of the staff should be involved in the countdown. An open house complete with refreshments and appropriate speeches should be held 1 or 2 days prior to the arrival of the first patient. Every effort should be made to encourage all of the hospital staff to drop by for the celebration. Frequently such openings are attended by upper and middle management, and the workers who will actually be involved in the day-to-day operation do not attend. This is unfortunate; to avoid its occurrence it may be necessary to use innovative methods of invitation.

The closer the opening date becomes, the greater the pressure to open early. Suddenly the institution that did not have such a unit will find that the patients are lined up awaiting admission. Do not capitulate! It is better to open as scheduled, prepared, than a day early, unprepared!

Throughout this book you will find references to the tendency for special care unit staffs to be estranged from the general unit personnel. It is not an easy problem to solve, nor is it unusual. If an ounce of prevention is ever applicable, it is in this situation. Try to make the new unit part of the hospital; start by keeping everyone informed of progress in construction, fund raising, hiring, etc. Post information on employee bulletin boards and use the hospital newsletter for a monthly update. Most important, all bulletins should convey the message that the unit belongs to everyone in the hospital.

The importance of the role of the medical director for specialty care units has been acknowledged by governing agencies, and it is expected that in the not-too-distant future some levels of critical-care units will be required to have a full-time, salaried, board-certified physician in charge. Presently, it is not unusual for a critical-care unit to have a paper director whose physical contact with the unit is limited. This precludes progress and stifles the creativity of the entire staff. It ensures that nurses' time will be spent in solving constantly recurring problems that should be the responsibility of the medical director. In a critical-care unit where the medical director is infrequently present, the nursing staff must decide on varying interpretations of the written policies. Admission and discharge decisions are often based on the power or popularity of the admitting physician rather than on patients' needs.

In Chapter 11, Kateri Heckathorn and Sharon A. Smith have written about management as it applies to nursing. Theirs is a realistic approach to the development of nurse managers, recognizing that the "Peter Principle" has long prevailed in the selection of nurse managers.

It is no less difficult for a nurse to become a manager than it would be for someone with a degree in business administration to become a nurse. They encompass two different bodies of knowledge and to some extent require different approaches to problem solving. These authors have recounted from their own experiences the steps necessary to accomplish creative and dynamic leadership. Management theory is available in numerous textbooks; however, few publications have applied it to critical care.

One management principle identified in Chapter 11 states that no person should be responsible for the supervision of more than ten people or report to more than one person. It is interesting to observe that the organizational structure of many nursing departments violates this principle. For example, the head nurse of a six-bed ICU with eighteen staff nurses, six aides, and two unit clerks may have no other leadership positions in the TO for that particular unit. Although the head nurse may assign a staff nurse to assume charge responsibilities for each shift, in effect, the head nurse is responsible for twenty-six subordinates. The product of a hospital should be patient care first and foremost. When does the head nurse have time for meaningful supervision? Can there be another business that pays so little attention to product supervision?

The head nurse must counsel and write a yearly evaluation for each member of the staff in addition to the daily tasks of management. Staff members expect and deserve the time for their head nurse to listen and discuss problems they may have. It is the head nurse who gives the most appreciated praise and likewise the most worrisome criticism. When the head nurse is responsible for twenty-six staff members and six patients as well as the coordination between physicians, allied health personnel, and other departments, is it any wonder that the stress levels escalate?

Since a critical-care unit is one of the most stressful work settings in health care, superior management skills are required at all levels of leadership. The ability to organize, communicate, and develop subordinates is acquired through education and practice. Critical-care nurses must insist on the opportunity and time to acquire managerial skills before accepting the responsibility of leadership positions.

CHAPTER 9

Recruitment and staffing

Jane M. Kahn

The main thrust in the development of specialty units came about in the early 1960s. These units generally consisted of cardiac monitors for patients suffering cardiac dysrhythmias. The creation of such units made it mandatory to develop specially trained nurses to manage these patients.

In 1963 the United States Public Health Service funded two such training proposals—one at Cedars-Sinai Medical Center in Los Angeles and one at New York Hospital/Cornell University Medical Center in New York City. During the 1960s the number of short-term general hospitals with critical-care facilities increased 440%.[1]

Critical-care units have been further delineated into specific units for respiratory, pediatric, neonatal, trauma, and shock patients.[2] This escalation in the number and types of units for the critically ill has created a massive problem in providing nursing staff for these patients.

In the majority of critical-care centers, it is the nurse, not the physician, who is responsible for managing a patient in crisis. And yet "almost ten percent of all professional nurse positions (defined to include unbudgeted positions) are unfilled and almost one-fifth of the hospitals state that twenty-five percent or more of their desired positions are not filled."[3]

IDIOSYNCRATIC CONSIDERATIONS

The idiosyncrasies of a given institution often determine the staffing needs of a particular critical-care unit. Before developing or redeveloping the staffing pattern for a specific critical-care unit, information about the community and the hospital in general must be gathered.

Information on the community should include the Bureau of Labor Statistics' data on ages, occupations, and incomes of the population. The data will show a direct correlation between the age of the populace and the type of health problems. For instance, more cardiovascular patients may be seen in a large geriatric population, whereas a community with many young families will require pediatric and trauma facilities.

Statistics on the classification of emergencies and distribution by days and hours can be obtained from the local fire and police departments as well as private ambulance services. This information will assist in staffing determinations as well as equipment preparedness.

After securing statistical data from community resources, gather information idiosyncratic to the institution. The most valuable data are available from the medical records department. Many hospitals use the Professional Activity Study-Medical Audit Program (PAS-MAP) system of data collection.[4] These data include number and types of surgeries, number of admissions from the emergency department to critical-care units, peak hours for critical-care admissions, and peak periods of high census in critical-care units.

Staffing in critical-care units is also affected by the support services. It is not only important to know the hours of service, but also to have a clear identification of their function. For example, does the respiratory therapy department perform arterial blood gas (ABG) tests on a 24-hour basis, or are they a nursing responsibility? These added or deleted tasks affect the staffing pattern. Consider the functions of the following departments:

1. Recovery room
2. Pharmacy
3. Biomedical engineering
4. Respiratory therapy
5. Laboratory
6. Secretarial personnel
7. Social worker/patient and family advocate

The following administrative factors directly influence critical-care nursing needs:

1. Admission and transfer policies
2. Complexity of procedures performed in the units
3. Use of standardized procedures
4. Affiliation with medical/nursing schools
5. Quantity and quality of nursing/medical supervision
6. Ratio of professional nurses to auxiliary personnel
7. Ratio of licensed nursing personnel to patients
8. Use of float or temporary nursing personnel
9. Required continuing education hours
10. Methods of record keeping
11. Legal constraints[5] (example 1, p. 124)

THE BUDGET

Fiscal allocations for critical-care units determine the development of a staffing pattern. A budget is "a format plan of future operations expressed in quantitative terms and serving as a basis for subsequent control of such operations."[6]

The nursing service budget must reflect departmental goals in number and type of nursing personnel and continuing education programs. The nursing service administrator must receive input from the financial managers as to the procedure for preparation, time periods covered (fiscal year), and formats designed. Personnel policies such as vacation time, illness, pay scales, pay increments, turnover percent, and statistics affect the preparation of a staffing budget.

Since the budget for critical-care areas constitutes a large portion of the overall nursing department budget, it may be advisable to form a critical-care budget committee. This committee should include leadership personnel as well as a representative from the finance department. The committee members who actually function in the critical-care unit provide direct input regarding patient care needs. Following are the purposes of the committee:

1. To review previous staffing and position allocation for safe and effective patient care
2. To review standardized procedures presently performed by nurses
3. To consider procedures that could be delegated to others
4. To consider the financial feasibility of implementing additional nursing responsibilities
5. To evaluate equipment that may increase or decrease nursing time
6. To recommend changes in organization and structure

The annual personnel budget is formulated on information gathered from these sources. Then, divide the fiscal year by calendar months or quarters and examine the activity levels during these periods. For example, the number of open heart surgeries may be highest in January and February and therefore require a 1:1 nurse/patient ratio. In this situation, the budget should project increased recruitment activity in the preceding quarter (October, November, December), allowance for overtime, and a decrease in vacation hours.

Thus, budgeting personnel for the critical-care units is a method of allocating human resources (nurses) to meet a goal (direct and indirect patient care). The nursing service administrator should receive monthly financial statements of expenditures and revenues, which should be shared with the leadership staff members responsible for controlling activities in the critical-care units. These individuals must account for the actual monthly performance compared with the budgeted resources.

Of the three major budget areas (personnel, supplies and equipment, and capital expenditures), accounting for human resources is the most difficult. Variations do not necessarily reflect poor budgeting decisions. Increased patient census, which will require increased nursing care hours, cannot always be predicted.

Since budgeting is a dynamic process used to plan and control activities, the entire budget should be reviewed at least every 6 months to more accurately analyze needs.

RECRUITMENT

Hospitals routinely advertise in local newspapers and nursing journals for personnel. This is not the only method to recruit qualified nurses. Other means include monetary rewards for referrals, participation in meetings and conventions, open-house programs, recruitment trips, and many other programs that enhance the hospital's reputation. The success of such programs is measured by the number of responses received for each dollar spent.

Recruitment depends on the philosophy of the organization. The first step to be determined is the type and extent of recruitment to be pursued. The budget can then be developed. Each institution must develop its recruitment budget based on the number of critical-care beds, the desired staffing pattern, turnover history, effective advertising media, travel and mailing expenses, and personnel costs. Data on terminations and overtime are the nurse recruiter's best armamentaria for justifying an adequate budget.

One must consider the behavioral components of recruitment. The nurse administrator must be cognizant of the fact that the individual who holds the major responsibility for securing critical-care nurses holds a key position in the organization. This person's knowledge must include, but not be limited to, licensure and legislative regulations, the community served by the institution, patient population, services provided, and the philosophy and standards of patient care. For critical care, the recruitment specialist must be able to readily describe levels of services, professional qualification requirements, educational and experience requirements, as well as the physical plant. Basically the recruitment specialist must be a salesperson, but must also possess communication skills, persuasiveness, and perhaps most important, a basic belief in the institution's philosophy and policies in caring for critically ill patients. It is much easier to recruit nursing personnel for a well-equipped, critical-care unit with 24-hour support services such as laboratories, an engineering department, and computerization.

The initial phase of recruitment consists of developing advertisements emphasizing the extrinsic rewards of the position. These extrinsic factors should include salary; insurance and retirement programs; vacation, holiday, and sick time; staff development programs; tuition reimbursement; interpersonal and/or social activities; housing; and geographical location. The extrinsic rewards can be communicated through various types of advertising media.

Recruitment based on the intrinsic rewards is far more complicated. However, the intrinsic factors such as professional growth, self-fulfillment, and independent practice opportunities are best communicated by critical-care staff members who have benefited from these advantages. These individuals know more about the milieu of their institution. By involving them in a recruitment incentive program, their enthusiasm can be directed to benefit the overall recruitment program.

Transferring nurses from within the institution to the critical-care unit can also be effective. A nurse who has demonstrated good medical/surgical skills and a desire to learn critical-care nursing is a valuable asset. This individual knows the institution and has been observed performing professional skills.

Selection process

The most important factor in staffing a critical-care unit is the selection process: finding the right person for the unit. The three major areas to consider in selecting a critical-care nurse for a hospital are interpersonal factors, educational background and experience, and technical qualifications. To evaluate technical qualifications, an applicant's education (including basic, advanced, and continuing) and experience in critical care must be reviewed. The educational background reflects the applicant's ability and motivation and may indicate career goals. The applicant's experience can be reviewed in terms of length of employment, type of facility, specific job functions, and reason for leaving. The interviewer can request permission from the applicant to secure references. Applicants without critical-care experience who request the specialty should be considered. Past experience and educational background may be identified with the objective of uncovering a potential trainee.

All applicants should be evaluated in terms of past achievements and aspirations that may give some indication of the individual's values, goals, and willingness to make a work commitment. The interviewer must assess the applicant's interest and motivation for caring for the critically ill, provide a job description, and carefully weigh what the position has to offer against the applicant's expectations.

An attempt must be made to determine the applicant's interpersonal relationships, emotional stability, and ability to function under stress. The applicant's social history (family and friends, hobbies, and interests) will indicate an ability to interact with others.

The initial interview may be conducted by the personnel department or nurse recruiter. The purpose should only be initial screening and reference checking. The critical-care nurse applicant should be interviewed by the supervisor or head nurse of the unit; this interview should include a tour of the facility.[7]

Testing mechanisms

Since the ideal personality profile for a critical-care nurse has yet to be identified, any psychological or personality testing is suspect and open to challenge. To date, most applicants are hired on the basis of the interview process. Tests to determine clinical knowledge and skills are the ideal methods for evaluating critical-care applicants. Presently, two testing methods are available: one is the examination administered by the AACN Certification Board. More than 3000 nurses have successfully completed the testing and are board certified in critical-care nursing (CCRN). Although it is unrealistic to require all nurses employed in critical-care units to be CCRNs, it is a goal for the future.

The second testing method is a written examination developed by each critical-care department. The examination should include the following sections:

1. Anatomy and physiology
   a. Cardiovascular
   b. Pulmonary
   c. Neuromuscular
   d. Renal/metabolic
2. Pharmacology
3. Special techniques (CPR, ABG, etc.)

The examination must be tested for reliability and validity. Although there are four major methods of determining reliability, the test-retest method is the most easily administered. "You produce the two sets of data by administering the instrument once (the test): then after some period of time, long enough to allow forgetting to occur but not so long that change would be expected, you administer the instrument to the same people a second time (the retest.)"[8] The data are considered reliable if results of the two sets of test scores correlate.

The difficulty in the test-retest method is determining the time interval between the tests. Turnover statistics may be most applicable in determining appropriate intervals. Generally, the retest should not be given less than 6 months or more than 1 year from the time of the original test. Rearrangement of the same questions is advisable to test knowledge rather than rote memory.

Validity refers to the testing tool itself; does it measure what it is supposed to measure: Are the questions relevant? The three basic methods for estimating validity of the testing tool are construct validity, concurrent validity, and predictive validity. Construct validity should produce gross differences for the same test delivered to two significantly different groups. For example, a critical-care examination given to a group of obstetrical nurses and a group of critical-care nurses should produce grossly different scores.

Concurrent validity correlates scores from a new tool with those of a pre-existing measurement. This method is acceptable only if the pre-existing measurement is valid and different from the current one.

Predictive validity is the most potent procedure. Data from the testing tool are used to make predictions about the behavior of respondents. It is this method that is widely applied in screening applicants for critical care. Follow-up on the predicted behavior is mandatory to ensure a close correlation.

In preparing test questions, it is imperative that they be general enough to have wide applicability. For example, a question referring to a technique peculiar to a specific institution or unit would be considered neither a reliable nor a valid test of the knowledge of critical-care nurses unfamiliar with the institution's idiosyncrasies.

Appropriateness is an essential characteristic for all test questions. Are the questions appropriate for a given set of respondents? The appropriateness of the testing tool is closely related to its validity.

Objectivity must be maintained throughout the testing phase. Objectivity can best be maintained by use of multiple-choice questions. Fill-in and essay questions require more subjective types of analysis or scoring.

After a satisfactory interview and screening process, carefully consider placement of the critical-care candidate. For example, someone with limited skills and experience should initially be placed in a telemetry or lower crisis–type unit in which the stress level can be managed. Malplacement of critical-care nurses is often the major cause of high turnover.

STAFFING PATTERNS

The development of staffing patterns and nursing care ratios received a tremendous amount of attention after World War II.[9] Today, the majority of acute care facilities use a patient classification system as a means of quantifying each patient's direct nursing care needs.

In adult critical-care units, the general method of staffing is a 1:2 ratio. The range often includes 1:1 ratios for open heart surgery and intra-aortic balloon assist patients and 1:3 in some cardiac care units unless otherwise stated by law.[5]

The general method of determining staffing needs is to project the average census for a given unit and the number of nurses needed on duty based on a 1:2 ratio. Although there are elaborate methods prepared to determine staffing formulas,[10] generally, 1.5 nurses are employed to keep one nurse on duty. This factor takes into account holidays, sick days, vacations, and regular days off.

Cullen and co-authors at the Massachusetts General Hospital use a scoring system based on the types of interventions performed in caring for the critically ill (example 2, pp. 125 and 126). Adaptation of the "Therapeutic Intervention Scoring System" (TISS) should include routine activities such as bathing and oral hygiene. The purposes of the TISS model are to:

1. Determine appropriate utilization of intensive care facilities at the Massachusetts General Hospital
2. Provide information on nurse staffing ratios for various patient care areas
3. Quantitatively validate a clinical classification of critically ill patients into four categories, thereby simplifying and organizing activities relating to patient care
4. Analyze cost of intensive care relative to the extent of care offered[11]

Although the TISS method serves to quantify interventions performed in critical-care units, it does not determine the qualifications of the nurse carrying out these interventions. Thus, ideal staffing includes matching the severity of the patient's illness with the skill level of the nurse.

The critical-care nurse can be categorized into levels, such as those developed by Weil and Shubin[2] and Kahn[12] for the Center for the Critically Ill.

The purposes for classifying critical-care nurses are as follows:

1. Allows the general medical/surgical nurse the opportunity to ease into the critical-care setting
2. Defines the position description for all levels
3. Forms the basis for curriculum development
4. Allows for promotion of nurses on the basis of their knowledge and clinical skills without promoting them into the administrative hierarchy
5. Defines the knowledge and skills required of critical-care in-service instructors
6. Classification is applicable to all institutions based on individual types, sizes, and technological support

The classifications listed have been modified to meet current standards of practice:

Critical-care nurse I

1. Minimum of 1 year general medical/surgical clinical experience
2. Successfully completed an approved course in critical-care nursing
3. Has mastered essential skills
   a. Basic dysrhythmia identification
   b. Cardiopulmonary resuscitation
   c. Care of patient on a mechanical ventilator

Critical-care nurse II

1. Met requirements of CCN I
2. Minimum of 1 year experience in critical care
3. Has evidence of fifteen educational contact hours a year in critical care
4. Has mastered intermediate skills
   a. Assists with insertion of arterial lines and cares for patient with arterial lines
   b. Draws blood gases
   c. Sets up and calibrates a pressure transducer

Critical-care nurse III

1. Minimum of 2 years experience in critical care
2. Passed the AACN Certification Board examination
3. Possesses sophisticated skills
   a. Performs a thermodilution cardiac output
   b. Cares for a patient with intracranial pressure monitoring
   c. Cares for a patient receiving intra-aortic counterpulsation balloon therapy

Despite all efforts to predict staffing needs for critical-care units, uncontrollable variables such as emergency admissions often alter these plans. Contingency plans should include the use of on-call personnel, part-time employees, or qualified agency assistance.

Retention

Retention of highly skilled critical-care nurses is often the key issue in staffing. Although a certain percentage of turnover may be considered acceptable (education, mobility, etc.), other causes may be traced to the high degree of stress placed on the critical-care nurse. Sources of this stress may be categorized as behavioral, technical, and organizational (example 3, pp. 126 and 127). Although these three sources are highly integrated, they do represent one method of approaching personnel crisis in critical-care units.

Nurses who enter the critical-care field do so with the expectation that they can enhance their professional roles through specialization. The critical-care setting allows the nurse to give total patient care. The very nature of these units requires the nurse to be technically competent. No matter how much time is devoted to the emotional support of the patient and family, the nurse is required to perform some tasks at regular and specific intervals, such as administering fluids, measuring central venous pressure and pulmonary artery wedge pressure, and drawing arterial blood gases. Frustration may easily develop for the nurse who views technical tasks as belonging to a subprofessional group. On the other hand, some nurses may receive their greatest satisfaction from maintaining a high degree of technical skill without much regard for personalized patient care. The resulting role conflict for these nurses is based on their inability to integrate technical and personalized patient care skills, because both are essential components of critical-care nursing.

Another area of stress is that of impending patient crisis and death. This inherent situation requires the nurse to constantly be prepared to provide life-support interventions as well as emotional support to the patients' families.

Some nurses suffer from isolationism because critical-care units are physically separated from other areas. Rarely do nurses from other areas enter these units. Social stigmas may result because of lack of knowledge of each group's role and function.

Conversely, an esprit de corps may develop within the critical-care unit, which may help to minimize turnover. Behavioral stress for the critical-care nurse can also be minimized by an available and skilled critical-care team. These resources are vital in providing security when medical and technical assistance is needed.

The automated world and technical advances are responsible for changing the role of nursing. These changes began in the early 1960s with the use of ECG monitoring devices. This approach to patient care was viewed negatively by some who felt their traditional roles would be interrupted. Others accepted technical advancement as a complementary element in the care of the critically ill. Nevertheless, the highly sophisticated technical world is all around us and demands our attention in relation to nursing personnel.

Nurses in critical-care environments are aware of the fact that electronic devices extend their precision in assessing patient conditions and in initiating immediate and reliable action during a crisis. These devices may serve as sources of security for some, or they may present a great deal of stress or anxiety to others. Different perceptions seem to stem from various areas. The first consideration is in the selection and purchase of various electronic devices. Unfortunately, in many institutions the physician, nursing administrator, and purchasing agent select the equipment. However, the team should include the staff nurse and biomedical engineer; they are the ones who use and repair the equipment.

Second, a thorough in-service program must be planned to allow the nurse to learn the use and care of equipment. These programs are more effective if the entire team (physician, nurse, and biomedical engineer) is involved. It is generally accepted that electronic devices are effective for patient care only if the critical-care staff can use them efficiently. The efficiency can be greatly enhanced if in-house personnel are available for training and troubleshooting rather than relying on the manufacturer's representative.

Although numerous organizational aspects affect the stress level of critical-care nurses (example 3, pp. 126 and 127), the flexibility of staffing patterns appears to be the most crucial. Special attention must be given to time off by arranging two days off together, long weekends, and approved absent days whenever possible. Some hospitals have initiated a 12-hour schedule of 4 days on duty followed by 4 days off duty. This program provides both continuity of care as well as sufficient time away for the nurse; therefore, it meets patients' and staffs' needs.

The critical-care staff should provide input into the scheduling, and the majority must agree to adhere to it to assure its effectiveness.

Example 1: TITLE 22: HEALTH FACILITIES AND REFERRAL AGENCIES[5]

70465. Coronary Care Service Staff

(a) A physician shall have overall responsibility for the service. This physician shall be certified or eligible for certification in cardiovascular disease by the American Board of Internal Medicine. If such a cardiologist is not available, a physician certified or eligible for certification in internal medicine by the American Board of Internal Medicine, with training and experience in cardiovascular disease, may administer the service. In this circumstance, a cardiologist, qualified as above, shall provide consultation at such frequency as to assure high quality service. The physician in charge shall be responsible for:

1. Development of a system for assuring physician coverage
2. Implementation of a system for assuring physician coverage
3. Conducting education programs in coronary care for physicians
4. Assuring there is a continuing education program for nursing personnel in coronary care
5. Final decision regarding admissions to and discharges from unit

(b) A registered nurse with training and experience in coronary care nursing shall be responsible for the nursing care and nursing management of the service.

(c) All licensed nurses shall have had training and experience in coronary care nursing.

(d) There shall be not less than two nursing personnel physically present in the coronary care unit when a patient is present. At least one of the nursing personnel shall be a registered nurse.

(e) The licensed nurse:patient ratio shall be 1:2 or fewer at all times. Licensed vocational nurses may constitute up to 50% of the licensed nurses.

70495. Intensive Care Service Staff

(a) A physician with training in critical care medicine shall have overall responsibility for the intensive care service. This physician or his designated alternate shall be responsible for:
1. Implementation of established policies and procedures
2. Development of a system for assuring physician coverage
3. Final decision regarding admissions to and discharges from the unit
4. Assuring there is continuing education for the medical staff and nursing personnel

(b) A registered nurse with training and experience in intensive care nursing shall be responsible for the nursing care and nursing management of the intensive care unit when a patient is present.

(c) All licensed nurses shall have training and experience in intensive care nursing.

(d) There shall be not less than two nursing personnel physically present in the intensive care unit when a patient is present. At least one of the nursing personnel shall be a registered nurse.

(e) The nurse:patient ratio shall be 1:2 or fewer at all times. Licensed vocational nurses may constitute up to 50% of the licensed nurses.

(f) An inhalation therapist, physical therapist, and other supportive service staff shall be available depending upon the requirements of the service.

Example 2: THERAPEUTIC INTERVENTION SCORING SYSTEM[11]

Four points
a. Cardiac arrest and/or countershock within 48 hours
b. Controlled ventilation with or without PEEP
c. Controlled ventilation with intermittent or continuous muscle relaxants
d. Balloon tamponade of varices
e. Continuous arterial infusion
f. Pulmonary artery line
g. Atrial or ventricular pacing
h. Hemodialysis in unstable patient
i. Peritoneal dialysis
j. Induced hypothermia
k. Pressure-activated blood infusion
l. G-suit
m. Measurement of cardiac output
n. Platelet transfusions
o. IABA (intra-aortic balloon assist)
p. Membrane oxygenation

Three points
a. Hyperalimentation or renal failure fluid
b. Pacemaker on standby
c. Chest tubes
d. Assist respiration
e. Spontaneous PEEP
f. Concentrated K^+ drip (>60 mEq/L)
g. Nasotracheal or orotracheal intubation
h. Endotracheal suctioning (nonintubated patient)
i. Complex metabolic balance (frequent intake and output, Brookline scale)
j. Multiple ABG, bleeding, and stat studies
k. Frequent infusions of blood products
l. Bolus IV medications
m. Multiple (>3) parenteral lines
n. Vasoactive drug infusion
o. Continued antidysrhythmia infusions
p. Cardioversion
q. Hypothermia blanket
r. Peripheral arterial line
s. Acute digitalization
t. Active diuresis for fluid overload or cerebral edema
u. Active Rx for metabolic alkalosis or acidosis

Two points
a. CVP (central venous pressure)
b. >2 IV lines
c. Hemodialysis for chronic renal failure
d. Fresh tracheostomy (less than 48 hours)
e. Spontaneous respiration via ET tube or tracheostomy
f. Tracheostomy care

One point
a. ECG monitoring
b. Hourly V.S. or neuro V.S.
c. "Keep open" IV route
d. Chronic anticoagulation
e. Standard intake and output
f. Frequent stat chems
g. Intermittent IV medications
h. Multiple dressing changes
i. Complicated orthopedic traction
j. IV antimetabolite therapy
k. Decubitus treatment
l. Urinary catheter
m. Supplemental oxygen (nasal or mask)
n. IV antibiotics

Example 3: CAUSES OF STRESS FOR NURSES IN CRITICAL-CARE UNITS

Behavioral
1. Integrative ability to combine technical and personalized patient care skills
2. Impending patient crisis and death

3. Needs of patients' families
4. Isolationism
5. Skills level and availability of the critical-care team

Technical
1. Selection and placement of equipment
2. Availability of biomedical engineer
3. Training in the use of equipment
4. Availability of supplies
5. Availability of allied specialists such as respiratory therapists

Organizational
1. Medical organization
2. Policies, procedures, protocols
3. Quality and quantity of nursing supervisory personnel
4. Flexibility of staffing pattern
5. Critical-care staff development

REFERENCES

1. The nations hospitals: a statistical profile, Hospital **44**:466-470, 1970.
2. Weil, M. H., and Shubin, H.: Introduction to symposium on care of the critically ill, Mod. Med. **39**:83, May, 1971.
3. Sloan, F. A.: The geographic distribution of nurses & public policy, Bethesda, Md., 1975, DHEW Publication No. CHRA/75-53, p. 86.
4. Summary of PAS reports: Commission on professional and hospital activities, Reprint 81, Ann Arbor, Mich., 1975, Commission on Professional and Hospital Activities (CPHA).
5. California Administrative Code, Title 22, Social Security Division 5, Licensing and Certification of Health Facilities and Referral Agencies, Calif., June, 1975. Published by Office of Administrative Hearing Department of General Services.
6. Seawell, L. V.: Hospital financial accounting theory and practice, Chicago, 1975, Hospital Financial Management Association.
7. Bermosk, L. S., and Mordan, M. J.: Interviewing in nursing, New York, 1964, The Macmillan Co.
8. Fox, D. J.: Fundamentals of research in nursing, New York, 1966, Appleton-Century-Crofts.
9. Shoemaker, N. J.: Application of modern management methods and operations research to nurse staffing patterns in the ICU. In Current Topics in Critical Medicine, vol. 2, 1977, Basel Karger Publishers, pp. 161-167.
10. Arndt, C., and Huckabay, L. M. D.: Nursing administration: theory for practice with a systems approach, St. Louis, 1975, The C. V. Mosby Co.
11. Cullen, D. J., et al.: Therapeutic intervention scoring system: a method for quantitative comparison of patient care, Crit. Care Med. **2**(2):57-60, 1974.
12. Kahn, J. M.: Trends in the educational process for the critical care nurse, Crit. Care Med. **3**(3):123-126, 1975.

BIBLIOGRAPHY

Alexander, E. L.: Nursing administration in the hospital health care system, St. Louis, 1972, The C. V. Mosby Co.

Arndt, C., and Huckabay, L. M. D.: Nursing administration: theory for practice with a systems approach, St. Louis, 1975, The C. V. Mosby Co.

Bermosk, L. S., and Mordan, M. J.: Interviewing in nursing, New York, 1964, The Macmillan Co.

California Administrative Code, Title 22, Social Security Division 5, Licensing and Certification of Health Facilities and Referral Agencies, Calif., 1975, Office of Administrative Hearing Department of General Services.

Cullen, D. J., et al.: Therapeutic intervention scoring system: a method for quantitative comparison of patient care, Crit. Care Med. **2**(2):57-60, 1974.

Cullen, D. J., et al.: Indicators of intensive care in critically ill patients, Crit. Care Med. **5**(4):173-179, 1977.

Fox, D. J.: Fundamentals of research in nursing, New York, 1966, Appleton-Century-Crofts.

Hariton, T.: Interview: the executive's guide to selecting the right Personnel, New York, 1970, Hastings House, Publishers, Inc.

Herman, S. M.: The people specialists, New York, 1968, Alfred A. Knopf, Inc.

The nation's hospitals: a statistical profile, Hospital **44**:466-470, 1970.

Kahn, J. M.: Trends in the educational process for the critical care nurse, Crit. Care Med. 3(3):123-126, 1975.

Kahn, J. M.: Administrative management of the center for the critically ill, Heart Lung 2(2):218-221, 1973.

Kellogg, M. S.: What to do about performance appraisal, New York, 1975, American Management Associations.

Koontz, H.: Appraising managers as managers, New York, 1971, McGraw-Hill Book Co.

Seawell, L. V.: Hospital financial accounting theory and practice, Chicago, 1975, Hospital Financial Management Association.

Shoemaker, N. J.: Application of modern management methods and operations research to nurse staffing patterns in the ICU. In Current Topics in Critical Medicine, vol. 2, Basel Karger Publishers, pp. 161-167.

Sloan, A.: The geographic distribution of nurses & public policy, Bethesda, Md., 1975, DHEW Publication No. CHRA/75-53, pp. 81-95.

Weil, M. H., and Shubin, H.: Introduction to symposium on care of the critically ill, Mod. Med. 39:83-85, May, 1971.

Weil, M. H., and Shubin, H.: Critical care medicine, New York, 1976, Harper & Row, Publishers, Inc.

Wiley, L.: Job evaluations: giving them and getting them—with less of a hassle, Nurs. '75 5(11):75-80, 1975.

CHAPTER 10

In-service training and continuing education

Kathryn M. Lewis

I remember reading somewhere that Thomas Paine once said, "These are the times that try men's souls." I cannot think of a more precise description of the feelings of the nurse who is responsible for developing and implementing the educational programs for a critical-care nursing staff. Each day of each week can bring new opportunities to provide dynamic educational programs for those nurses responsible for maintaining proficiency at the bedside of the critically ill patient. Educators may sigh in relief, realizing they are not alone; creative, but perhaps unfulfilled ICU nurses may tend to point their fingers; and health care administrators probably wish those units would just go away. The burden of providing a sufficient number of adequately prepared critical-care nurses is never-ending in most institutions. At times, the demand can overtax the faculty and educational facilities.

Managers of general units are frequently resentful when a large portion of the educational budget must be expended for ICUs, because in many hospitals the funding of critical-care units comes from the overall nursing budget. Anyone who is associated with critical-care nursing appreciates the fact that the needs are indeed greater, but one must also accept the necessity of justifying the educational programs. This is not to say that general units do not appreciate the scope of patient care and subsequent need for high-level education. Certainly they, too, must document their needs, and often general medical and surgical units reflect high-priority care. Critical-care managers and educators, by virtue of patient acuity, require greater numbers of professionally educated nursing staff members. They must then assume the responsibility to provide documentation supportive of those needs.

The methods and scope of education for the critical-care staff sets those nurses apart from the general schema. However, in most hospitals critical-care in-service training is part of an overall educational program, supported from the general education fund and answerable to nursing and hospital administration. Therein lies the problem of being different! Let's face it, the way in-service training is handled for all staff nurses does not always fit the needs of ICU nurses. Their training covers more material, in greater depth, and has greater patient implications. Valid documentation of learning needs is often overlooked. This handicaps hospital and nursing administrators who make funding decisions. Providing this documentation is the responsibility of criti-cal-care managers and educators. If we say we need it, we should provide data to support the need and show its use.

The justification for documenting need lies in the fact that critical-care nurses accept responsibility for precise and rational decision making in a life-support situation on a daily basis. They must be ready, alert, and prepared to make sound judgments based on current information. These nurses have changing values and are not satisfied being one of the crowd. They resent being identified solely with the mechanization that makes up a good part of their environment. They are creative, anxious, and enthusiastic. But they get burned out, become frustrated and, oh yes, they admit to "being dumb" about a lot of things. One can say they work there because they want to, so they can leave anytime. This is true, but if they did leave, who would defibrillate the coronary patient, dialyze the renal patient, make medication decisions based on electrolyte balance and blood chemistries, maintain important hourly as-sessments, and prevent chaos by anticipating patient problems and coordinat-ing the intervention?

Management and education must keep up with these nurses and their needs. It would seem that a substantial outlay is needed to protect the invest-ment made to recruit, hire, and train critical-care nurses to function in a highly sophisticated, high-priority unit. Often when educational needs are not met, nurses leave and the process starts all over; the unit becomes unstable, morale is down, cooperation is minimal, assessments are slipshod or harried, in-travenous infusions are unrecorded, equipment is misused, and medication errors are made. Worst of all, patients suffer.

Indeed, there are many reasons for providing educational programs specific to critical care. These include physician dissatisfaction, patient com-plaints, labor costs that are excessive in comparison with other nursing facilities, greater evidence of hazards to patients and staff, waste of time and materials, and errors in care and judgment.

An educational program will not be the final answer to all these problems. However, a strong program that is responsive to patient needs, as well as those of nursing, can alleviate many of the difficulties. Although most health care administrators recognize critical-care needs as being greater in scope and in-tensity, they often lack clear-cut, nonemotional evidence that the investment is justified. The need is for a practical educational program built on patient need, which rationally considers the cost of human and material resources. Following are the foci for discussion in this chapter: to provide guidelines for planning and developing programs of orientation and continuing education, and to provide the manager with the background necessary to make an informed decision regarding the critical-care areas.

ORIENTATION: DEVELOPING DECENTRALIZED IN-SERVICE RESPONSIBILITY

In 1975 a research study was completed to describe the purpose, organization and approach to orientation and continuing education in thirteen hospitals.[1] The study highlighted and supported the benefits of decentralized staff-faculty responsibility. In this approach, one instructor is responsible for nurses in a group of units referred to as a clinical service. This method is a unique approach to the task of providing education for all areas and especially critical care.

In this system, faculty members are responsible to the director of education and in turn to the nursing administration. Faculty members plan and implement specific orientation activities and follow-through for new employees. In addition, programs for continuing education are usually planned and implemented for employees on their work shift. These efforts involve identification and coordination of priorities for each group of units.

The instructor works closely with each coordinator (head nurse) to determine priorities for activities, expected standards of care, and knowledge and skills expected of each nurse. Faculty members are not in line positions and this contributes to comfortable working relationships with coordinators as well as staff members. This system can be adapted in any institution and benefit general units as well as critical-care units. The advantages are as follows:

1. Instructors are used efficiently throughout a clinical service.

2. Continuity of education and experience is provided for the orientee when a specific instructor, clinically proficient in that area, is available.

3. Continuing education programs are more practical, specific, and realistic.

4. Orientees are better prepared, thus more secure.

Staff instructor orientation

To provide relevant and accurate teaching and to remain active clinically, instructors should be required to maintain direct clinical involvement in the service to which they are assigned. This is imperative in critical care. The advantage is that the instructor is constantly aware of the patient profile and changing needs of the nursing staff. Instructors plan their own schedules, focusing around orientees and educational activities, while allowing time for bedside clinical practice. One instructor works a full day every 2 weeks, whereas another works a full week every 3 months at the bedside to provide similar exposure to current patient and nursing needs.

An active personnel department that uses an employee relations expert can provide the instructor with up-to-date information on duties and obligations of employees and their accountability. Often, rulings in employee management hearings are made based on the presence or absence of educational documentation. It is important to remember that legally, if it is not written, it is not so. Therefore, what was taught and when it was taught must be documented.

The instructor contributes to the management decisions made by the coordinator through anecdotal records, counseling, and comments on supervised tasks. All of this takes time, skill, and a thorough knowledge of policy and procedure. These skills are vital when developing methods of documenting educational programs and skills practice.

Developing a format for orientation and continuing education

Perhaps the most important task in developing a relevant orientation program is identifying the specific patient profile. From this information nursing functions can be outlined. Requisite knowledge, skills, nursing decisions, and tasks can be enumerated. The educator then develops the teaching-learning experiences necessary to provide the background for sensible and accurate nursing intervention.

Another approach is to develop a survey, allowing the staff to outline their general and specific expectations. Open-ended statements or questions will elicit more information. The survey might begin by asking for a description of the patient profile. A sample survey follows:

> The patients we care for are usually . . .
> I feel most inadequate . . .
> Is there a routine or standard of care for your patients? yes____ no____ If yes, is it written? yes____ no____
> Available to the staff? yes ____ no ____
>
> If the nurse makes any decisions/observations regarding admission and/or discharge from your facility, what criteria does she use to help with the decision?
>
> Is it written? yes____ no____ How often is it used?
>
> The tasks I do every day include . . .
> I most want to learn about . . .

Knowing the patient profile gives the educator insight into the academic background and skills required of the staff nurse for patient care. The nurse making crucial decisions must know the related anatomy and pathophysiology; disease entity; expected therapies; and relevant observations, assessments, and interventions. This knowledge should be documented as behavioral objectives from which a general lesson plan can be developed. If a nurse comes to the unit knowledgeable in these areas, validation must be based on the completion of the behavioral objectives. In any case, teaching and validation should be done, using a skills list for resource and documentation.

Developing the skills list

The skills list should be developed according to the activities expected of a nurse in a specific unit. Following are characteristics of the skills list:

1. Reflects the tasks performed
2. Provides documentation of performance and/or knowledge of concepts
3. Consistently used for all nursing employees
4. Requires an objective method of measurement (standards) and the re-test frequency acceptable for safe practice
5. Requires an observer who knows the standards as well as the skills to be assessed

One specific and important advantage of the skills list is that it makes possible a systematic appraisal of each nurse's proficiency based on objective criteria. The skills list can help identify tasks everyone must learn and perform to maintain effective practice. It can also help establish the content of instruction needed to enable the person or group to reach or maintain a higher than adequate level of job performance.

To review current skills lists or develop a new one, an inventory should be developed, itemizing various nursing tasks and/or knowledge. An example of an inventory follows:

ACTIVITY	FREQUENCY OF PERFORMANCE			
Inhalation therapy	Always	Freq.	Occa-sionally	Rarely
1. Nasal cannula	☐	☐	☐	☐
2. Oxygen tent	☐	☐	☐	☐
3. MA-1 ventilator	☐	☐	☐	☐
4. Servo-ventilator	☐	☐	☐	☐
5. Engström ventilator	☐	☐	☐	☐

Once basic tasks are reviewed, more in-depth knowledge can be assessed.

	Required	Desirable	Not necessary
A. Neurological evaluation			
1. Assess level of consciousness	☐	☐	☐
2. Know signs and symptoms of increased intracranial pressure	☐	☐	☐
3. Perform basic reflex testing:			
a. Grips	☐	☐	☐
b. Wrist extensors	☐	☐	☐
c. Babinski's reflex	☐	☐	☐
B. Cardiovascular evaluation			
1. Identify dysrhythmias			
a. Sinus	☐	☐	☐
b. Atrial	☐	☐	☐
c. Ventricular	☐	☐	☐
d. Blocks	☐	☐	☐

One approach is to list items according to systems. Other tasks, including the use of specific electronic equipment, can be categorized accordingly. Once noted, the usefulness of the data for future planning and development is obvious. All the surveys will be invaluable in developing the final skills list.

Reviewing a skills list. The skills list should be reviewed yearly to keep it current and to adequately reflect tasks being done. Also the terminology should be examined carefully; it should enhance the statement so that specific objectives can be defined as met, or the deficiency identified. For example, the following phrases are specific enough to reflect objectives that are met: "demonstrate how . . ."; "describe three configurations . . ."; and "enumerate steps in . . . ." When practical application is difficult to appraise, then phrases such as, "statements made reflect knowledge of . . . ," can be used.

Whatever phraseology is chosen, the list must be used consistently. Commentary should be brief, objective, and signed. To be valid, the skills list should be reviewed with the nurse, a documentation of learning activity (practice, patient care, etc.), a documentation of on-the-job performance, completed within a specified length of time, and kept in the employee's file.

Although the educator and nurse complete the documentation, the coordinator is ultimately responsible for its review, completion, and authorization of need for retraining. The coordinator also retains the responsibility for reviewing the skills list to verify that it reflects the skills and knowledge necessary for safe practice in the specified area.

Accountability. Once the skills list has been in use, it can be used to document hours of classtime, practice, or other related activities. Table 4 shows the completed core orientation program, noting content, activity, and rationale as planned with the ICU coordinator.

Table 4. Special care unit(s) guidelines for LPN and RN orientation

Content	Activity	Rationale
Initial interview New employees, Mon. afternoon	Identify role of staff faculty	Employee needs to know expectations, plans, objectives
Transferring employees, as scheduled (can be done prior to actual orientation) Lasts from 30 min-1 hr.	Identify processes of orientation, objectives and content; refer to initial orientation packet	Process of orientation can accelerate depending on validation of employee's present knowledge and skills; employee must be able to identify rationale and do procedures
Orientation calendar	Review orientation calendar	One week of orientation is done on shift
		Employee, staff faculty, and responsible coordinator will have copy
		Employee will know what is planned; may be able to prepare with independent study
	Emphasize that orientation is considered probationary	Identify progress employee makes; coordinator and/or supervisor are kept informed

Table 4. Special care unit(s) guidelines for LPN and RN orientation — cont'd

Content	Activity	Rationale
	Explain preceptor system	RN will be preceptor; information as to ability level of orientee discussed with supervising nurse; feedback shared and documented
	Explain use of examinations	Exams help in planning; they are not pass/fail; they indicate nurse's strengths and areas of need
General orientation	External cardiopulmonary resuscitation (ECPR): practice with mock codes; bagging Policy and procedure review Equipment review Body mechanics Chart forms and charting exercises Legal aspects of charting Kardex Medication review	Provide class and related practice; note on skill lists appropriate date and time (when formal class times are complete, skill lists are kept in skill list book in each nurses' station; orientee can record name of patient and date procedure was carried out)
Specific orientation activities	Tracheostomy class (2 hr plus practice) Chest drainage systems Intravenous therapy, admixture, blood administration, heparin lock (2 hr plus practice)	
RN leadership skills	Two days of class with assignment	Provide experience and class content relative to RN roles, resource, techniques; knowledge necessary for RN in leadership role
Medication examination	Examination	Provide tangible information validating present knowledge of medications and administration of medications and intravenous infusions Serves as basis for further teaching-learning Provide tangible information validating present knowledge and skill of patient care policies
Philosophy and policies of special care unit facility	Review from orientation manuals; discussion follows (1 hr)	Employee needs to know that it is not enough to know how to do procedure; special care unit nurse must know norms,
Concepts of critical-care nursing	Discussion and examples	implication, priorities, plan of care; must be able to explain physiology in brief terms, identify what can happen next, and what role will be

Continued.

Table 4. Special care unit(s) guidelines for LPN and RN orientation—cont'd

Content	Activity	Rationale
Basic electrocardiography	See lesson plans: review and validation (2-6 hr): full course (44 hr)	Provide class, and related experience and practice Orientee should be able to explain complexes and/or dysrhythmias in terms of what is happening in heart, where can it lead, what does patient look like; focus is nursing implication and priorities; it is not enough to identify dysrhythmia by name
Reviewing drugs used for special care unit nursing	Discussion of drugs: see lesson plan for specific assignment Provide handouts on specific drugs: introduction to emergency medicines; guidelines for giving intravenous medicines	Orientee should be able to explain use of each drug in terms of why, how, when, maximum/minimum dose, implications
Arterial lines and central venous pressure (CVP)	Setup and practice (2 hr)	Nurse should be able to set up pressure line and monitor; define acceptable patient parameters; troubleshoot equipment malfunction; identify waveforms and implications
Peritoneal dialysis	Audiovisual aid and practice; see lesson plan and practice on charting (1 hr)	
Congestive heart failure; pulmonary edema	See lesson plan: practice rotating tourniquets as well as with machine (1 hr)	Nurse should describe signs and symptoms of left- and right-sided failure
Processes of observation, assessment, planning	Class discussion led in direction of problem-oriented care and modified problem-oriented charting (2 hr plus practice)	
Neurological assessment	See lesson plan (1-2 hr)	
Cardiac assessment	See lesson plan (1-2 hr)	
Prefilled syringes	Practice	
Cannula care	See lesson plan (1 hr)	
Care of patient with chest tubes	Class plus practice (1 hr)	Nurse must organize approach to patient-centered care with priorities in critical-care nursing
Intubation	See lesson plan and procedure manuals ($\frac{1}{2}$ hr)	
Gastrointestinal intubation		
Defibrillation and cardioversion	See lesson plan: demonstration on unit (2 hr)	
Acid-base balance and hypoxia	See lesson plan (2- to 3-hr classes)	
Care of patient receiving ventilation therapy	See lesson plan (2 hr)	
Respiratory review	See lesson plan (1 hr)	
Heart sounds	See lesson plan (1-2 hr)	
Intracranial pressure	See lesson plan (2 hr)	
Thermodilution	See lesson plan (2 hr)	

Table 4. Special care unit(s) guidelines for LPN and RN orientation — cont'd

Content	Activity	Rationale
Arterial monitoring techniques; drawing blood from arterial line	See lesson plan (2 hr plus practice)	Nurse must organize approach to patient-centered care with priorities in critical-care nursing
Monitoring techniques with transducers	See lesson plan (2 hr plus practice)	
Hypothermia	Audiovisual aid and lesson plan (1 hr)	
Pacer	Class demonstration, exam (1 hr)	
Swan-Ganz catheters, thermodilution	Class demonstration, exam (2 hr plus practice)	
Patient care experience	Hands-on care usually with supervision	Nurse should be able to discuss patient's condition, problem for that day, identify priorities in care; charting should be objective, concise, problem-oriented in approach
	Initially, observation and assistance; no charting	
	Patient care progresses with supervision as does charting process	
	See lesson plan	
Evaluation		Glean appropriate feedback; assess program content
Final interview	Interview with coordinator	Document experiences; one copy kept in orientee's file; one copy kept in staff development office

This plan is also in effect for coronary care and neurological intensive care. Variations are made according to specialty. For example, the coronary care nurse would not be expected to learn the process and procedure of invasive intracranial pressure monitoring. However, if rotation to that area were to be planned, the class and practice would be available on a continuing education basis.

These classes carry the American Nurses Association (ANA) Continuing Education Units (CEUs), which are an added benefit and incentive.

Planning orientation

Part of the hiring process includes the completion of a form (Fig. 10-1) reflecting the nurse's clinical experience, as well as the usual information about professional and academic background. The personnel interviewer is the first person to scan the information and determine if the applicant meets the standards set by the clinical coordinator of the patient unit for which the nurse is applying. If the information is verified and a clinical coordinator is interested, an interview is scheduled.

The information serves as a screening device and saves the coordinator time, since only prospective employees who meet the qualifications and standards for employment in that unit are interviewed.

	Unit assigned _____
	Employment date _____
	This space for interviewers use only

1. Name _____
   Last   First   Middle

—————————————If you are hired, this information will be used to plan your orientation—————————————

2. Job title (circle):   3. RN's and LPN's: Arizona license no. _____ Expiration date _____

   RN   LPN   NA   Orderly   Technician   Temporary permit no. _____ Expiration date _____

4. Type of basic program (circle one): Assoc. Degree Diploma Practical Nurse Baccalaureate Nursing Assistant Course Service Experience

5. School of nursing: _____   6. Year of graduation _____

7. Location of school _____

8. Education beyond basic program: _____

9. Have you had a course in pharmacology? Yes _____ No _____

10. Nursing experience: _____
    a. New graduates—state name, location, and size of the hospital and agencies where you had your student clinical experience.
    b. Experienced graduates—state name, location, size of hospital or agencies, position held, and length of time in position.

11. Have you had other hospital experience (volunteer, other department technician, etc.?) If so, what was it and for how long a period of time?

12. Have you worked:	Never	A few times	Many times	(For "many times", what was your status?)
A full eight-hour period				
Evenings				
Nights				
Weekends				

13. What is the greatest number of patients you have taken care of or been responsible for? _____

14. Which methods of providing nursing care are you most familiar with? Functional _____
    Group nursing _____ Team nursing _____ Other (please state) _____

15. Have you had leadership preparation? As a student: Classes _____ Experience _____
    As a graduate: Classes _____ Experience _____

16. Have you had experience working with:	Yes	No
a. House medical staff (interns, medical students)		
b. A ward or unit management system		
c. The metric system (cc, g, etc.)		
d. Administration of medication to a group of patients		

If you answered "yes" to "d" please respond to the following: How many patients? _____
How many times? _____

Fig. 10-1. Data sheet identifying past nursing experience.

The coordinator discusses items of specific interest, relating the applicant's patient care experience to the unit's patient profile. In-depth discussion can provide insight as to the similarity of the applicant's past experiences and current unit practices. This kind of information is shared with the instructor, so that orientation activities can be planned to avoid redundancy. This will maintain a high interest level and allow more time to be spent on individual needs, whether in the classroom or at the bedside.

The form was designed by clinical coordinators, and items and terminol-

17. Have you had experience in:	No	Yes	How long?	Status		No	Yes	How long?	Status
Cardiology-medical					Newborn nursery				
Cardiology-surgical					Obstetrics-postpartum				
EENT					Oncology (cancer)				
Emergency department					Operating room				
General medical					Orthopedics				
General surgical					Outpatient department				
Geriatrics					Pediatrics				
Gynecology					Premature nursery				
Intensive care					Public health				
Kidney center					Recovery room				
Labor and delivery					Rehabilitation				
Mental health					Respiratory				
Metabolic					Urology				
Neurology					Other (specify)				

For RNs and LPNs only:

18. Please check the appropriate spaces indicating your experience status for the skills listed below.

	Never	Once	Few times	Many times	Need experience		Never	Once	Few times	Many times	Need experience
CVP readings						Medication administration					
Cardiac monitors						Nasopharyngeal suctioning					
Cardiopulmonary resuscitation						Pacemakers					
Chest tubes						Patient assessment					
Dialysis-peritoneal						Referrals-hospital resource people					
Dialysis-cannula						Referrals-community health agencies					
Dressing change-nonsterile						Respirators, use of					
Dressing change-sterile						Rotating tourniquets					
Evaluation of personnel						Staff assignments					
Hypo/hyperthermia treatments						Stoma care					
Insertion of retention catheter						Stryker frame					
Intravenous therapy: starting						Teaching patients					
regulating						Tracheostomy care					
adding medications						Tube feedings					
Irrigations: catheter						Writing: care plans					
nasogastric tubes						discharge summaries					
wound						nursing histories					
Isolation						Other:					

Comments:

Signature of applicant

Signature of interviewer

Date

Fig. 10-1, cont'd. For legend see opposite page.

ogy were agreed on by them, so that all levels of patient care are reflected. As a result, specific information can be sought for all types of patient care profiles. A copy of this form is retained in personnel, and another shared with the clinical instructor.

Orientation calendar. Once the core is devised the master calendar should be developed. An example of a single week in such a plan is given on p. 140.

ORIENTATION CALENDAR FOR 1 WEEK

Monday

8 AM-12 PM	General orientation, benefits, fire safety
12-1 PM	Lunch
1-2:30 PM	ECPR, bagging, mock code practice
2:45-4:30 PM	Procedure and policy review

Tuesday

7-9 AM	Body mechanics with practice
9-10 AM	Equipment review
10-12 PM	Legal aspects of charting, chart forms, practice
12-1 PM	Lunch
1-2 PM	Intake and output and graphic charting
2-3:30 PM	Medication review

Wednesday

7-9 AM	Care of patient with tracheostomy
9-10 AM	Chest tubes
10-12 PM	Intravenous infusion class (includes infusion pumps, blood administration, tour of pharmacy, code cart)
12-1 PM	Lunch
1-3:30 PM	Assessment

Thursday

7-9 AM	Breath sounds class with AV and practice
9-11 AM	Medication assignment review
11-12 PM	Lunch
12-1 PM	Pacers
1-2 PM	Review philosophy, skills lists, etc.
2-3:30 PM	Tour unit

Friday

7-9 AM	Review and practice with monitors, lead placement, cardioversion, defibrillation
9:30 AM	Meet with ICU pharmacist
10:30 AM	Meet with respiratory therapist
11:30 AM	Lunch
1-3:30 PM	Tour; check carts ad lib

Times are planned to allow maximum coverage of a topic. In the event a nurse is knowledgeable in the topic, the time will be spent in the unit in clinical practice.

Preceptorship

On some occasions the nurse orientees relate only to the instructor. To avoid this, the educator should provide learning situations in which employees relate to the persons in charge of the unit, emphasizing that the instructor is not the only resource person available.

However, there are instances, particularly when a new, inexperienced employee must learn a great number of tasks and skills under the direction of the instructor, that a dependent relationship may occur. This should occur rarely, and joint counseling efforts between the employee, coordinator, and instructor will usually correct the problem. A preceptor concept minimizes the chance of this problem occurring.

Preceptorship should not be frightening; it simply means people helping people. When a nurse has particularly good skills and an interest and ability to teach, it is advantageous to buddy a new nurse with her. Preceptors (sponsors or buddies) should be rewarded verbally, as well as with consideration at merit evaluation time. Preceptors expend considerable effort and assume a great deal of responsibility. These special people should be developed in terms of teaching-learning theory, as well as their own specialty. In certain instances a licensed practical nurse (LPN) will be a preceptor to a registered nurse (RN) orientee. This is not unusual, since the preceptor should be chosen and developed in terms of ability to teach, support, and guide another staff member. The preceptor should be patient and honest, remember what it is like to be new, be willing to suggest repeat classwork and more practice if indicated, and maintain adequate documentation.

The concept of preceptorship augments the general supportive climate of the team effort in critical care. All team members can and should be encouraged to help with teaching. In that way, no one individual becomes all things to all people. The coordinator should be involved in teaching in the classes or clinical areas; respiratory therapists are excellent sources of information, support, and instruction; and social workers can help identify psychosocial problems encountered in the ICU. In one unit the senior respiratory therapist assumes responsibility for working with the staff in orientation and continuing education. The causes of respiratory failure, care of the ventilated patient, and blood gas interpretation are discussed. The nurses are given an opportunity to breathe on a ventilator with and without positive end expiratory pressure (PEEP). The biomedical engineer and a group of clinical instrumentation specialists teach classes in monitor techniques, concepts of arterial monitoring, and thermodilution cardiac output. These specialists also function at the bedside, assisting nurses and physicians in the many invasive monitoring procedures.

The intensive care pharmacist meets with the new staff, explains the innovation of the ICU satellite pharmacy, and is available to the orientees, as well as the staff, on a continuing basis. The pharmacist participates in bedside rounds, contributing the appropriate expertise.

In addition, the instructor for the acute and chronic kidney centers assumes the responsibility for teaching the care required by those patients. This team approach is dynamic and satisfying in maintaining the strength and resources of a critical-care unit. The team approach is vital, and the people most involved are the ones who make it work.

It should be noted that during orientation new personnel are not included in the count in planning staffing for several days. This allows them freedom to work without stress and the flexibility to leave the unit for formal classtime without jeopardizing patient care.

A nurse might well complete orientation in less than the maximum time allotted. However, a new graduate or a nurse without previous ICU experience may require much more in terms of support as well as classtime. Should a nurse require additional education or extension of orientation, the need must be documented by the instructor and the nurse. The coordinator then considers the request before it is submitted to nursing administration for approval.

Should a nurse require disciplinary action of any nature, it is documented by the instructor and/or coordinator. When the instructor does not function in a line position, and the coordinator retains the ultimate responsibility for decision making, there is more consistency and less confusion about leadership. This should not imply that the instructor does not become involved in the correction process; however, when improvement is not evident, the coordinator is responsible for final decisions.

Throughout orientation the nurse is expected to supplement the program through self-study. This provides reinforcement of new information and adds to requisite knowledge. The concept of home study is thought to develop the habit of reading and research throughout the nurse's career, which is especially important for a critical-care nurse.

Low ebbs of disinterest and a feeling of being overwhelmed are to be expected. Support, patience, and learning incentives help prevent such occurrences from leading to apathy. Management may accomplish this by offering support verbally and at merit time. Also, a coordinator could ask for specific help on a project of special interest or in problem solving. Sending the staff nurse to conferences is most valuable. Of course, a commitment to share knowledge should be made and followed through on return from the educational program. The educator can assist by providing information on how to attend a conference, what to expect, etc. Many people have never attended a workshop or conference, and when confronted with a program offering concurrent educational tracts, they can lose valuable time trying to figure out where to go and when.

Classroom vs. clinical learning

Much of what the critical-care nurse learns at the bedside are skills based on requisite knowledge accumulated over time. The nurse has completed a program of academic study and brings good basic knowledge that can be enriched with bedside experience; patient + disease + intervention should = recovery. In fact, most of us remember the course of disease, treatment modalities, and results from patients we have cared for. This does not alter the fact that many bedside judgments are based solely on clinical learning from the classroom or some form of self-study. The current surge in accurate nursing history and complex assessment skills makes it imperative that the nurse absorb textbook information as well as clinical norms and deviations. For example, the nurse must synthesize information relating to anatomy and pathophysiology, the anticipated response to specific medication therapies, what invasive monitoring values really mean, how they should be interpreted, and how this information can alter a care plan. The nurse must also know what additional interventions, if any, should be anticipated and what should be deleted.

Although the core orientation program provides a maximum of 60 hours in class, the activity allocation during those hours makes the difference. Planning patient care responsibilities as an adjunct to current topics being covered in class is a valuable tool.

Classroom theory. This chapter does not include details on techniques of classroom instruction; many bibliographic references cover this topic. Please note, though, how necessary it is to provide for creativity in the classroom. Active nurses get bored very easily sitting in class, particularly when it is only review and reinforcement. Class content needs to be structured in such a way that the teacher can determine what the group knows, build on it, and introduce new material.

For example, some method should be used to evaluate current knowledge on a topic; such a tool is the pretest. This may be considered threatening to some but by titling it review or exercise, such stress may be avoided. Once completed, it can be used as a teaching tool, reviewing and enlarging on important facts noted in the format. The student's pretest need not be graded but the results can be used for future class content and/or patient care activity.

The concept of grading should not be taboo. In more formal classroom activity, pass/fail is mandatory to measure compliance with written behavioral objectives. For example, an ECG, pharmacology, or acid-base determination course must be graded. A passing grade of 80% may be considered unrealistic, but health care professionals have the responsibility to use this new information in helping a patient's recovery; therefore, stringent criteria are indicated.

Group participation should be encouraged in class. Activities should be used that will enhance students' ability to work together. Game theory is a valuable asset to accomplish learning that can be tedious no matter what the approach. Programmed instruction using branching and scrambling devices seems to be most successful.

At any rate, the nurse educator should take time to plan an activity that will generate interest and participation. It may take a bit longer to devise than the tried and true lecture methods, but results can be outstanding and long remembered.

Time, place, equipment. Although the core orientation provides all the class time within 10 days (the orientee is not included in the staffing count), the coordinator and educator can plan a feasible schedule providing bedside experience as well. Administrative support of the educational program is a must.

Class should be held away from the unit to avoid distraction and interruptions. Often the 5-minute walk to class allows a breather, a separation from the clinical area, and a chance to prepare mentally for classroom activity. The environment should be comfortable, clean, well ventilated, and never crowded. Classes can be as short as 20 or 30 minutes. It is important to preserve interest and enthusiasm and have the learners leave discussing the session and looking forward to the next class.

Various audiovisual aids (AV) can be used (slides, films, filmstrips), but at no time should any presentation be done without introduction, commentary, and/or free discussion afterward and practice when appropriate. The poor use of AV materials seems to stem from the fact that many educators expect the program to do everything and answer all questions. An AV program reinforces and brings to light confusing thoughts and questions. It should be a kickoff for discussion and practice. Handouts and guidelines should be developed, highlighting the series and perhaps presenting a few questions to be answered. When a particular presentation is outdated, discuss why it was done that way and why the change was made.

Most university libraries have access to the National Library of Medicine's computerized on-line information system. A simple terminal linked to the main computer memory can request information at anytime with immediate results. This system can provide the instructor with a current source of information.

MEDLINE cites recently published articles on specific biomedical subjects whereas AVLINE contains references to audiovisual instructional materials in the health sciences. All audiovisual items have been professionally reviewed for accuracy, currentness of subject content, educational design, and technical quality. AVLINE can save time for the instructor looking for audiovisual materials on a specific topic. The alternative to AVLINE is reviewing materials oneself. Here is an example of a computer willing to work for nursing and not asking to be taken care of itself.

One method that could be used prior to class, especially with learners of varying backgrounds would be to have them complete the following statement: the one real question I want answered in this program is . . . .

These statements are filled out anonymously, shared with the group, and class discussion and responses are encouraged. This exercise is particularly helpful during difficult learning modules in which learners are not too secure with the previous class activity. Responses from the group generate discussion, and group learning occurs.

Team vs. the individual. By now it is apparent that participative learning should be encouraged. As a method developing shared learning and decision making, it supports the team approach to care. This is not to imply that there is never room for the individual, but occasionally better decisions can be made by a team. This team approach is sometimes difficult in critical care. An example of a very real problem is the in-command physician who competed to get into medical school, then competed to survive and stay in, and competed to set up and maintain a successful practice. Now the physician is asked to function on a team to share, compare, and work with others and their opinions. This will probably be a difficult transition. If the critical-care nurse realizes this, it may help avoid frustration. Tactful discussions will do more to develop team spirit and mutual support than toe tapping, mumbling, or shrieking. Trust, tact, honesty, and humor are the cornerstones required for team development.

The resource teacher. To be clinically competent and academically prepared does not ensure the ability to teach anymore than it ensures the ability to manage. When choosing a resource instructor, consider clinical expertise but also consider if the resource person is able to impart knowledge. Are objectives clearly defined? Are they specific and in writing? Does the resource person know what is expected for the particular unit? Is responsiveness to learners present? Is evaluation ongoing regarding carry-over of learning to the unit and patients? Is documentation complete, accurate, and timely?

Evaluation

Feedback is another often forgotten or ignored part of education. Fig. 10-2 and p. 147 represent evaluation forms given to nurses at the completion of class and/or orientation. The forms are reviewed, and adjustments are made based on staff suggestions. Effective use of the evaluation form depends on the following:

1. Assure confidentiality
2. Design questions that are brief and to the point
3. Allow some free response
4. Ask for suggestions
5. Allow the learner to complete the form in private, perhaps away from the classroom
6. Allow the learner to return the form within a period of time

Evaluations should be reviewed and discussed with the leadership staff. Changes in program can be decided by this group based on a report including objectives, plan, materials required, cost, and justification.

Summary

In summary, an orientation/continuing education program for a critical-care nursing service should be developed to meet specific patient profiles. It should provide a flexible approach to meet the needs of individual nursing staff members, regardless of academic background and clinical expertise. In developing such a program, documentation of patient needs, related skills, and procedures should occur. Methods used to meet the curriculum will ac-

Please circle the number above the most suitable comment. Use numbers 2 and 4 for "in-between" judgments. Leave question blank if you have no opinion. Ratings conscientiously and honestly given can be of great value to the instructor.

1. Do you find this course to be valuable in improving your competence in your present or future work?

5	4	3	2	1
Extremely valuable	Moderately valuable			Not valuable

2. Do you feel that the course is contributing to your education in general?

5	4	3	2	1
Very much	To a moderate degree			Not at all

3. What is your feeling about the amount and difficulty of the workload?

   a. In reading: Too much _____ About right _____ Too little _____

   b. In written work: Too much _____ About right _____ Too little _____

4. Were there opportunities for students' questions?

5	4	3	2	1
Questions often permitted		Questions sometimes permitted		Few questions permitted

5. Were the explanations of the instructor clear to you?

5	4	3	2	1
Very clear	Sometimes not clear			Often unclear

6. Were you stimulated to do your own thinking?

Yes _____ No _____

7. What is your impression of the way the instructor scheduled and planned her instructional material?

5	4	3	2	1
Very well planned	Moderately well planned			Poorly planned

8. a. Which one(s) of the classes were the most meaningful for you?

   b. Which one(s) were the least meaningful?

9. Do you have additional comments?

Fig. 10-2. Form used to evaluate ECG course.

cumulate and develop into a data source that is supportive of time, equipment, and resources vital to maintaining expert nursing care.

DEVELOPING A CONTINUING EDUCATION PROGRAM

Once the critical-care nurse is comfortable with the unit, patient care, rotation plan, etc., another task faces the educator, that of providing dynamic and practical programs for continuing education. Maintaining the interest and enthusiasm of the nursing staff while meeting their needs and those of the patients are accepted overall goals. How to accomplish these goals remains clouded in terms of topic selection, release time, place, and teachers involved, how often, and how long. It is like planning orientation all over, but in a more flexible manner. The methods discussed can be used for the individual nurse with a particular need, special care unit, and community.

RATING SCALE EVALUATION

Instructions: Please check the column below the rating that most accurately describes your evaluation of each class.

	Excellent: *I learned a great deal*	Well done: *I learned a good deal*	Just fair: *I learned a few things*	Poor: *I learned nothing*
Physical assessment	☐	☐	☐	☐
Breath sounds	☐	☐	☐	☐
Head-neck surgery	☐	☐	☐	☐
Care of the patient with tracheostomy	☐	☐	☐	☐
Ocular plastics	☐	☐	☐	☐
Respiratory therapy	☐	☐	☐	☐
Esophageal speech	☐	☐	☐	☐
EENT projects	☐	☐	☐	☐

Please leave this form with the instructor at the end of the day's activities.

The nurse with a problem

The approach to extending orientation in special individualized circumstances has been previously discussed. In addition to the orientee, who may need more time and effort to develop skills and/or clinical judgment, there is the experienced nurse who is noted to have a deficiency in some area. Occasionally this discovery comes about when an error in judgment, medication, omission, or commission occurs. Through discussion, the educator and coordinator should mutually agree on a plan and the allotted time release. Once this has been defined, the educator can meet with the specific nurse and plan the content, approach, and time. The need for cooperative planning is imperative because the nurse may often view the effort as a penalty for not knowing. This may occur regardless of a supportive environment. The cooperative participatory approach is valuable in overcoming this obstacle to learning.

Occasionally the need can be met by classwork, bedside preceptorship, or additional readings. Once the objectives and plans are decided, they should be documented and signed by the nurse, instructor, and coordinator for acceptance. In this way a contract exists for the investment in time, effort, and materials. The individuals also need to decide on a method of evaluation, especially if visible improvement is a stated objective. Documentation of the transaction from onset to evaluation should be done and included in the nurse's file.

GUIDELINES FOR ORIENTATION TO SPECIAL CARE UNIT(S)—CALENDAR OF ACTIVITIES

Monday	Tuesday	Wednesday	Thursday	Friday
5/2 7 AM E.R., "Seizures" 3 PM E.R., "Seizures"	**5/3** 7:30 AM D4, rec. room, "Special Procedures Cart" 7:45 AM E4, Dr. Cohen 3:30 PM E4, lounge, "Sexuality, No. 7, Homosexuality"	**5/4** 7:30 AM E5, "Special Procedure Cart" 2:15 PM E4, lounge, "Sexuality, No. 7, Homosexuality" 3:30 PM D4, rec. room, "Special Procedures Cart"	**5/5** 6-7:15 AM, 2:15-3:30 PM, 10-15-11:30 PM C3, ICU, "Peege" (film and discussion) 3:30 PM E5, "Special Procedures Cart"	**5/6** 8 AM E4, lounge, "Sexuality, No. 7, Homosexuality"
5/9 8 AM E4, lounge, "Peege" (film)	**5/10** 7:30 AM Rec. room, "Antihypertensives," Chuck Berry, R.Ph. 7:45 AM E4, Dr. Cohen 3 PM E.R., "Chest Tubes"	**5/11** 3 PM D4, rec. room, "Antihypertensives," Chuck Berry, R.Ph.	**5/12** 7 AM E.R., "Chest Tubes" 7:45 AM, 2 PM, 3:30 PM, 10:15 PM, 11:45 PM C3, ICU, "Isolation, No. 2," Mrs. Johnston 2:15 PM E4, lounge, "Peege" (film)	**5/13** 7:45 AM E5, "Isolation, No. 2," Mrs. Johnston 3:30 PM E4, lounge, "Peege" (film) 3:30 PM E5, "Isolation, No. 2," Mrs. Johnston

5/16	5/17	5/18	5/19	5/20
8 AM E4, lounge, "Assessment of Abdomen, Auscultation and Palpation" 2:15 PM, 3:30 PM, 10:15 PM C3, ICU, "Assessment of Abdomen"	7:30 AM D4, rec. room, "Regional Anesthesia," Dr. Sadler 7:45 AM E4, Dr. Cohen 3 PM E.R., "Antihypertensives," Chuck Berry, R.Ph.	7:45 AM E5, "Antihypertensives," Chuck Berry, R.Ph. 3 PM D4, rec. room, "Regional Anesthesia," Dr. Sadler	7 AM E.R., "Antihypertensives," Chuck Berry, R.Ph. 2:15 PM E4, lounge, "Assessment of Abdomen" 3:30 PM E5, "Antihypertensives," Chuck Berry, R.Ph.	3:30 PM E4, lounge, "Assessment of Abdomen"

5/23	5/24	5/25	5/26	5/27
2:15 PM C3, ICU, "Potpourri Renal Failure and Dialysis," Sherry Rhone, RN 3 PM E.R., "Care of Patients with AV Fistula," Sherry Rhone, RN	7:30 AM Rec. room, "Review of workshop" 7:45 AM E4, Dr. Cohen 8-9 AM,* 1:30-2:30 PM,* 4-5 PM,* 9:30-10:30 PM† "Crime Resistance Task Force, Self-Protection Classes" *Sexson Hall Lobby †Dining Room 6	7:45 AM, 2:30 PM, 3:30 PM E5, "Isolation, No. 2," Mrs. Mildred Johnston 3 PM D4, rec. room, "Care of Patients with AV Fistula," Sherry Rhone, RN 3:30 PM, 10:15 PM C3, ICU, "Potpourri Renal Failure and Dialysis," Sherry Rhone, RN	8-9 AM,* 1:30-2:30 PM,* 4-5 PM,* 9:30-10:30 PM† "Crime Resistance Task Force, Self-Protection Classes" *Sexson Hall Lobby †Dining Room 6	7:45 AM, 3:30 PM E5, "Isolation, No. 2," Mrs. Johnston

THOUGHT FOR THE MONTH: *The quality of your nursing care reflects your image!*

When the program may be the problem

There are occasions when a nurse or group of nurses become dissatisfied with particular aspects of the environment. Often these are manifested in complaints about working conditions, rotations, physician idiosyncrasies, and of course, salary. When complaints are directed at the educational program, the instructor and coordinator must be ready for honest self-examination. Despite planning, surveying, and analyzing, if staff members do not see relevance and are not interested, the programs are useless. One method of prevention is to provide a variety of programs, using different methods of approach and a wide variety of resource persons. Despite the size of the institution, the latter can be a problem. When few resource persons are available for programs, or are unavailable for all shifts, one approach is to suggest that a shift representative attend and function as reporter. The reporter should be acknowledged for the effort, but not overused, so others may also become involved.

Timing. There should be an effort to provide continuing education on shift, the advantage being a captive audience. The greatest disadvantage is not being available to all shifts at all times. However, the use of 10-hour rather than 8-hour shifts allows for periods of overlapping staff coverage. Then while one shift cares for the patients, the other shift can attend a class and then switch. This system has increased attendance, while reducing stress and distraction. The instructor must be able to manipulate orientation activities and planned in-service training around the clock and still manage to survive. The advantage to 24-hour scheduling is the flexibility and exposure to the entire staff. The disadvantage is the endurance required of the instructor.

One problem to be considered with on-shift programs is length. They should not exceed 40 minutes, 30 minutes plus time for seating, questions, and return to duty. Classes should be repeated frequently to reach maximal numbers of personnel. This method makes it easier to provide coverage for patient care.

The greatest disadvantage is having to cancel the program because the patient load is so great that coverage would be inadequate if some staff left the unit to attend. For this reason, many units not using the 10-hour shift prefer to have class just prior to or just after the shift. The nurses feel less anxious, since they are not leaving patients, thus they are more open, receptive, and less distracted.

The unit staff can choose the time appropriate for the majority, or a workable alternative may be offered by the instructor. An example of a continuing education program for various units in a critical-care clinical service is given on pp. 148 and 149. In this approach, the same topic is repeated three times for maximum exposure and availability. Class members get credit for attending on their own time. Some hospitals pay the employee for the hour of education. When this is not possible, the attendance performance should be recognized at merit time. Either way, the management and educators should support a personal commitment by the critical-care nurse to develop and grow.

Content. Many pharmaceutical and biomedical supply companies provide listings of audiovisual and printed materials available for continuing education. They are usually good quality and of no cost to the hospital. The material should be previewed prior to distribution and as always, the savings documented for budget purposes.

Handouts should be provided for all audiovisual materials, identifying the points to remember. Nurses cannot be expected to take notes because this distracts from the program content. As with any program format, a bibliography or a related article should be distributed for further study.

As in orientation, resource persons should be chosen with care. Since most continuing education classes are short and to the point, a team conference or case study is another approach. A member of the nursing and/or physician staff should be encouraged to develop the format, present the material, and again, distribute a related article. Pharmacists are excellent sources of information, and, as drug therapy becomes more involved, the need for continual updating is imperative.

Physician resources are important in planning, as well as implementing continuing education. Occasionally problems arise when they are late or cancel, but usually the risk is worth it. Ask the physician speaker to have an alternate in case cancellation is a possibility. It is advisable to always have a backup ready when speakers are scheduled. Also an emergency box containing an extension cord, extra projector bulbs, a hemostat for retrieving 35 mm slides stuck in the carousel, chalk, an eraser, and a pointer will be handy.

Interviewing physicians to determine educational needs from their point of view and to identify subjects they are comfortable teaching is a valuable time investment. These activities should be done regularly, not just when there is a physician complaint. Knowing the physicians, what they have to offer, and how they can be used contributes to the program. They are a part of the team effort and are generally appreciative and proficient.

Equipment. The 35-mm slide projector, screens, 16-mm sound and overhead projectors, and tape recorder are basic to most programs. Videotape recorders (VTR) are expensive but may be justified in the long run. With VTR, care in planning and production should include attention to objectives, the plan, and the presenter. The advantage is the reality of the program and the ability for repetition at any time and any place it is needed. As with other investments the number of showings and number of learners should be documented to justify the expense.

Community involvement

Hospitals within the community should be able to share their ideas, materials, and programs in an effort to maintain costs. In one community, representatives of the in-service departments of several hospitals meet periodically to share information, solve problems, and generally help each other with the processes involved in maintaining orientation and continuing education programs.

The critical-care nurses in each community should establish and maintain a local chapter of the American Association of Critical-Care Nurses (AACN). Each educator and member should become involved with planning and implementing programs of interest. Education committees for the chapter in Phoenix developed a program based on needs of the community. To be sure the program was realistic, practical, and of general interest, a survey was done throughout the membership. Altogether, there are many forms of needs analysis surveys (Fig. 10-3); one in particular lists possible topics of interest and information such as site selection and time of class. In this way convenience of the majority of potential learners is provided. The survey can also provide information about the profile of interested learners and can be distributed in the local critical-care chapter monthly bulletin with the following introduction:

Dear Critical-Care Nurse:

The education committee is in the process of planning to meet your special educational needs. Our objective is to help you keep abreast with current critical-care practices. We hope to do this by presenting a semester course in critical-care topics through the Community College District. Each topic will include a review of anatomy and physiology, pathophysiology, assessment, diagnosis, and nursing intervention as it is applicable and necessary.

It is *vital* to the preparation of such a course that we hear from you. What topics are you interested in? Is this a practical way to meet your educational needs? Your answers to these questions will be appreciated.

Please return this questionnaire in the enclosed, self-addressed envelope. We will report the results to you at the next few local chapter meetings.

Thank you,

The Education Committee

Providing a stamped envelope is not only a convenience to the recipient, but an added incentive to cooperate. In one instance the committee had an 89% response.

As with any other program, objectives must be specified, teaching-learning methods decided, and evaluations developed. Resources throughout the community should be used. Often groups tend to rely on one or two major institutions for speakers and hardware, but all efforts should be made to increase the scope and exposure to as many qualified speakers/teachers as possible.

Hospitals should support activities of local chapters as an added benefit and resource to continuing education programs. Meeting places and hardware should be made available on a rotating basis. Since most educational programs are held during off hours, educational facilities and/or meeting rooms are more

Please check one

Age group: 16-25 yr _____   Position: Head nurse _____
                    26-35 yr _____   Ass't head nurse _____
                    36-50 yr _____   Staff nurse _____
                    51-65 yr _____

Position: CCU _____   Number of years in this position
          ICU _____   Less than one _____
         NICU _____   1-3 _____
     Other _____   4-7 _____
                        10-15 _____

Last level of education completed   Hospital at which you are now employed
Diploma _____   _____
Associate _____
Bachelor's in Nursing _____
Master's in Nursing _____
Other _____

Transportation
Do you drive to work: Yes _____ No _____
If yes, approximately how many miles round trip? _____
If no, do you bike _____ bus _____ car pool _____ walk _____

Time and place
Please list your preference by numbering 1-4 (1 = 1st choice)
Central Phoenix _____   9 AM-11 AM _____   Other _____
Glendale area _____   11 AM-1 PM _____
Scottsdale area _____   1 PM-3 PM _____
Tempe area _____   4 PM-6 PM _____

Topics of interest

	Most interested	Maybe	Least interested
Metabolic crises			
Thyroid storm			
Adrenal crisis	_____	_____	_____
General assessment			
Lung scan			
Heart sounds			
Breath sounds	_____	_____	_____
Fluid and electrolytes			
General management			
Overdose			
Burns	_____	_____	_____
Blood replacement			
Therapy	_____	_____	_____
Crisis intervention	_____	_____	_____
Hemodynamic monitoring			
Swan-Ganz			
Arterial lines			
Cardiac			
CVP	_____	_____	_____
Neurological assessment	_____	_____	_____
Crisis in hematology	_____	_____	_____
Drugs:			
Antihypertensives			
Code arrest drugs			
Antibiotic therapy	_____	_____	_____
Burns	_____	_____	_____
Crisis in GI system	_____	_____	_____
Crisis in GU system	_____	_____	_____
Social diseases			
VD, alcoholism	_____	_____	_____
Cultural influences in critical care	_____	_____	_____
Legal aspects	_____	_____	_____
Diagnostic techniques			
Radiological findings			
Special procedures	_____	_____	_____

Are you interested in registering for such a course? Yes _____ No _____

Fig. 10-3. Needs analysis survey for continuing education. (Courtesy Greater Phoenix Area Chapter, American Association of Critical-Care Nurses.)

available. This courtesy to chapter membership is good public relations and supports the overall commitment to educating the people responsible for patient care in the ICU in any community hospital.

CONCLUSION

Hospital in-service training has been around a long time. Nursing in-service training has been around even longer, but decentralization of in-service training for critical care is new and vital. Regardless of the organization, learning will take place all the time. The decisions are: What kind? Is it good or bad? How much? How little? Why or why not? Quality patient care should be more than lip service for public relations and the JCAH. It should be a focus and a by-product of an investment made to give the best possible tools to nurses responsible for patient care and a dynamic and responsive educational program based on patient needs.

Nursing care reflects the image of the hospital, unit, and nurse. Why not make the effort to develop and maintain that image in the most responsive and responsible way known—it may even save a life!

REFERENCE

1. Innovations in inservice: decentralized staff faculty, Tempe, Ariz., 1975, Arizona State University.

BIBLIOGRAPHY

Argyris, Co.: Management and organizational development, New York, 1971, McGraw-Hill Book Co.

Benathy, B.: Instructional systems, Belmont, Calif. 1968, Fearon Publishers, Inc.

Eckleberry, G. K.: Administration of comprehensive patient care, New York, 1971, Appleton-Century-Crofts.

Espick, J. E., and Williams, B.: Developing programmed instructional materials, Belmont, Calif., 1972, Fearon Publishers, Inc.

French, W., and Bell, C. H., Jr.: Organizational development, Englewood Cliffs, N.J., 1973, Prentice-Hall, Inc.

Gorman, A. H.: Teachers and learners, Boston, 1974, Allyn and Bacon, Inc.

Gronlund, N. E.: Constructing achievement tests, Englewood Cliffs, N.J., 1968, Prentice-Hall, Inc.

Hudak, C., Gallo, B., and Lohr, T.: Critical care nursing, Philadelphia, 1973, J. B. Lippincott Co.

Johnson, S. R., and Johnson, R. B.: Developing individualized instructional material: a self-instructional material in itself, Palo Alto, Calif., 1970, Westinghouse Learning Press.

Kahn, J. M.: Trends in the educational process for the critical care nurse, Crit. Care Med. 3(3):123-126, 1975.

Knowles, M.: The modern practice of adult education, New York, 1970, Association Press.

Kron, T.,: Communication in nursing, ed. 2, Philadelphia, 1972, W. B. Saunders Co.

Leonard, G. B.: Education and ecstacy, New York, 1968, Dell Publishing Co.

Luft, J.: Group processes: an introduction to group dynamics, ed. 2, Palo Alto, Calif., 1970, National Press Books.

Mager, R.: Preparing instructional objectives, Belmont, Calif., 1963, Fearon Publishers, Inc.

Munch, J., Ed.: Units for special care nursing, Nurs. Clin. North Am. 7:311-395, 1972.

Popham, W. J., and Baker, E. L.: Systematic instruction, Englewood Cliffs, N.J. 1970, Prentice-Hall, Inc.

Smith, R. M.: Participation training, Adult Leadership 18:77-78, Sept., 1969.

Sulkin, H. A.: Some considerations in choosing training methods, Adult Leadership 15:98-101, Sept., 1967.

CHAPTER 11

Management

Kateri Heckathorn and Sharon A. Smith

Seemingly endless publications, workshops, and consulting firms are available to the beginning or seasoned manager looking for new and better techniques of management. This chapter is not designed to provide management theory. It translates management theory for practical application in various intensive care settings. The guiding premise is that management must be people oriented.

> The asset which towers above all others in business is not money, not buildings, not land, but men. Men inspired by confidence in one another. Men who see their own successes in the success of their business associates. Men who are not working for one another, but with one another.
>
> Money is not, and never can be, the one principal object of our business. We place the greatest stress and give the foremost place to the training of men and the giving of service. This is the business insurance of producing producers. The essential duty of the manager is clear. He becomes a manager not alone because he gives evidence that we can trust him to conduct the affairs of a store, but, beyond that, because he has proved to us that he can build another man to take his place. Once a business is wise enough to do this, the financial income of that business is assured.*

This quotation illustrates that the critical foundation of any effective organization is people. An effective organization is one with good team spirit, turning out high quality work that others talk about, copy, or envy. It is always developing new tools that make the work smoother, easier, or better and is constantly designing teaching programs to increase its workers' depth of knowledge and skill. An effective organization serves as a resource to others.

What makes it work? Some might believe it is a dynamic leader who generates ideas, policies, procedures, and programs that are effective, stimulating, and motivating. Certainly such a leader might have good ideas and pro-

---

*From *Main Street Merchant* by N. Beasley. Copyright © 1948. Used with permission of McGraw-Hill Book Co.

gressive programs, but if it is a one-man show, the organization is not going to be strong. It will lack the key element of an effective organization—team spirit.

Others might feel that an effective organization is just a matter of luck. It received all the committed, enthusiastic people who are full of creative ideas. Other divisions or units complain that they cannot attract that type of individual. It seems unfair that they should all be in one place. However, the fact is that in every group a wealth of human resources is waiting to be encouraged and developed. The effective manager knows people and their potential. By developing individuals and working through the group, the manager strengthens the organization.

Another statement that people often make about an effective organization is that it does not have to cope with the problems others do: lack of administrative support, power struggles between various groups, conflict over space, budgetary constraints, apparent lack of qualified people to fill staff or leadership positions, young inexperienced workers who seem to think the world owes them a living, or simply too much work with too few people to do it. No matter how effective an organization appears on the surface, it has problems to cope with and resolve. Some problems are unique to the setting; others confront all of us. Things that are advantageous to a small organization may cause problems in a large enterprise and vice versa. Problems and conflicts cause headaches, but they also stimulate change and growth in the effective organization.

The key to an effective organization is managers who are able to develop and use all the people within the organization to achieve organizational goals. Anyone within the organization who is responsible for the work accomplished by others will have to take on this managerial function. As the manager moves up the organizational ladder, more emphasis must be placed on developing and caring for people within the organization.

The focus of this chapter is the development of an effective nursing organization. The size of the organization does not matter; the same basic steps need to be taken regardless of an organization's size. The principles of management highlighted in this chapter will be supplemented with actual examples from the clinical setting to emphasize the efficacy of a planned, consistent approach to the management of a critical-care nursing service.

HOW TO START

Chances are you were appointed to a leadership position because you were a clinical expert in your unit. You were constantly rewarded by physicians and nurses for your insights, sound judgments, and nursing actions. Typically, most executive promotions are filled from within an organization, and managers are often chosen because of their technical rather than managerial competence. The assumption that a good staff nurse makes an excellent head nurse is a non sequitur unless managerial potential is present.

If as a new leader you continue to restrict your focus to clinical problems rather than extending your concern to include the management and development of others, your managerial effectiveness will be compromised. It has now become your job to take care of the staff so that they can effectively take care of patients. As a new manager you will be given a grace period, a kind of honeymoon at first. It is essential during this time to get to know staff members as individuals, sorting out their strengths and weaknesses, recognizing what special qualities each person has to offer. Take time to listen, ask questions, observe, and seek opinions as to future direction and possible changes. Search for ways to use your managerial strengths for the benefit of others and to establish trust, which is the foundation for mutual goal-setting.

It has been said that if you do not know where you are going, you probably will not get there. It is important to develop a philosophy and determine goals and objectives for the area before you can begin to accomplish anything. This philosophy serves as the foundation for the goals and objectives on which the organization will function. Following are essential steps for creating an effective organization:

1. Philosophy
2. Goals and objectives
3. Organization
   a. Organizational chart
   b. Job descriptions
   c. Selection of leaders
   d. Use of personnel
   e. Use of space
4. Communication
   a. Written communication
   b. Regularly scheduled meetings
   c. Committees
5. Staff development
   a. Orientation and continuing education
   b. Evaluations

These areas should be considered in sequence, although they may not be accomplished in sequence. The individuals involved will vary according to the size of the undertaking. In a small unit these steps might be best developed by involving the nursing staff of the unit. In a larger setting with several units, it might be more appropriate to involve the leadership personnel in developing the overall foundation and framework.

To best illustrate the actual implementation of these steps, the dynamics of a developing critical-care nursing service as it really began to work will be described. The process shows the mix of plans, people, and problems that evolved as the organization became more effective. As with any developing service, the realization of goals was marked by some successes, some near misses, and some failures.

The chairman of the newly created intensive care nursing service (ICNS) was hired from the outside by the director of nursing to be the nursing administrator and coordinator of a cluster of ICUs. Each unit was unique in purpose, background, and direction. Fortunately, the new chairman inherited a service that had superb medical care, a dynamic and supportive nursing director, an exceptionally qualified nursing staff, and capable young supervisors who were open and ready for change. This is not always the case for a new leader. If these advantages are lacking, it will be necessary to deal concurrently with clinical, day-to-day problems as well as organizational development. It is still possible to accomplish goals; it will just take longer.

Philosophy

Recognizing one's personal philosophy of management is the initial step in the planning process. The newly appointed chairman possessed a background in nursing administration. She did not pretend to be clinically competent, nor did she feel it absolutely necessary. Her philosophy was take care of your people and they'll take care of the patients. She defined her role as threefold: to help set directional goals for the ICNS, to act as a change agent in residence, and to develop and support the critical-care staff.

The philosophy of the ICNS evolved during frequent meetings with the supervisors who were responsible for the individual units. Although in the beginning it did not always seem relevant or exciting to the supervisors, the philosophy was written. In the process, a sense of purpose and togetherness developed. The philosophy is as follows:

> The Intensive Care Nursing Service is primarily concerned with creating an atmosphere where dignity and respect is maintained for each individual patient, his family, and all members of the health care team.
> A highly specialized, skilled, caring, and enthusiastic multidisciplinary team, with special resources at its disposal, provides close observation and critical-care nursing for postoperative patients and/or patients with serious chronic conditions.
> Qualities of caring and commitment are vital to the maintenance of the high standards of nursing practice which are necessary for the promotion of the health and well-being of all patients.[2]

Goals and objectives

Initially, a list of common problems within the units and possible approaches was compiled. Goals and objectives were slowly hammered out, and priorities were set. The result of this problem-solving approach was a concrete plan of action. However, the most important offshoot was the eagerness of the staff within each unit to write their own goals and objectives and set priorities. Once the staff got interested and involved, things began to happen. It has been said that if you can get 60% committed to change, you can swing anything! Certain goals were accomplished quickly, others moved slowly, some have not yet been accomplished. The overall objectives of the ICNS were refined to the following:

To promote an atmosphere where education and healing combine with re-
spect for the dignity of the persons served and serving.
To promote growth in responsibility for oneself and others and a sense of
shared responsibility for the larger institution.
To promote sensitive concern for the patient and his family.
To promote integrity in management and to provide efficient and economical
administration of human and technological resources.
To foster a climate which encourages freedom, creativity, and initiative.[3]

Organization

Organizational chart. Things that often seem so simple and clear-cut can be
the most confusing. One of the most incredibly simple and confusing is an organizational chart. Before drawing an organizational chart, ask the staff to
make a chart that illustrates the present nursing structure as they perceive it.
If the charts show even two different organizational patterns, it will be clear
why lines of command and communication are so important.

Managers should have no more than ten persons reporting directly to
them, and each person should be directly responsible to only one person. Informal lines of communication and authority must channel in the same direction and to the same person as with formal lines. Every staff member needs to
understand the difference between line and staff relationships; line means direct authority and responsibility, staff refers to collaborative relationships. A
title per se is not as important as the job itself. Never confuse the staff by calling persons by the same title if their functions are not the same in all units.
Horizontal or vertical lines, concentric circles, squares, or triangles may look
attractive, but unless all individuals can identify themselves on the organizational chart, it will not work.

A dynamic service will need to review and revise the organizational chart
at least annually. The ICNS organizational chart of relationships is shown in
Fig. 11-1.

Job descriptions. Job descriptions should be so clear that if the titles were
erased, staff members would recognize the description of their role. Samples
of job descriptions are available in a variety of places. It is helpful to look at
different formats, but never simply copy one. It is sometimes helpful to have
each category of personnel in the service write their own job description.
Then review it with the group, editorializing and refining it, but never adding
or subtracting parts. Drafts of trial job descriptions may be tested for a time to
be sure they include essentials. Job descriptions need not be written in stone.
An opportunity to expand or change the role can be a challenge. Yearly reviews and/or revisions are a necessity as the needs of the unit change.

Selection of leaders. When the organizational chart and job descriptions
are completed, the next important step is to choose and/or develop leaders
who can help you attain your goals. Your personal philosophy of life, strengths
and weaknesses, and style of leadership will be the deciding factors in choosing leaders. If the chemistry is right, people can work together despite differences in temperament, abilities, and experience. People need people to help

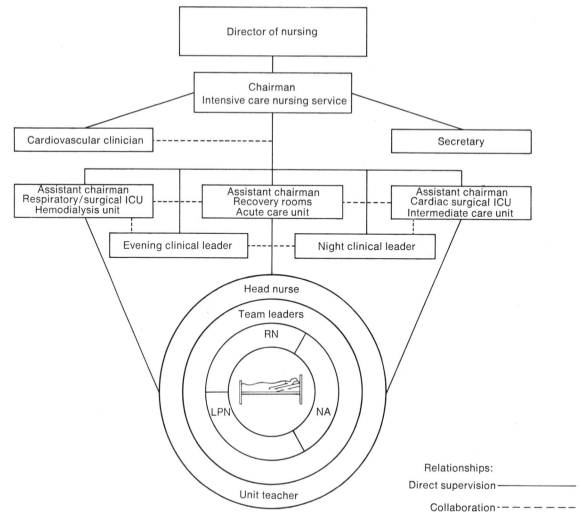

Fig. 11-1. Intensive care nursing service table of organization. (Courtesy Massachusetts General Hospital Department of Nursing, Boston, Mass.)

fill in their gaps. Two truisms of management are: no one can do everything alone, and no one of us knows as much as all of us. To be strong one must share. Therefore the selection of key people for an organization is critical. Not everyone has leadership potential, although most people believe they do.

The selection of leaders is an awesome task. The ICNS was fortunate to have an established departmental method to follow. Position openings were posted, and interested applicants completed resumes and listed their personal goals and objectives. Interviews were conducted by a small committee composed of specialty-oriented staff nurses and nurses already in similar leadership positions. The committee conducted objective interviews. Following are some of the questions asked of candidates for leadership positions: Are you effective in difficult circumstances? Do you develop subordinates? Do you get along with people? Can you accept change and conflict and enjoy managing it? Are you realistic? Are you willing to take risks and live with the consequences? Are you intelligent and aware of your strengths and weaknesses? Are you able to listen and make sound judgments? Are you self-confident? Are you naturally optimistic? Because happiness is an inside job and not a company responsiblity, leaders are needed who can set a positive tone for the staff.

Educational background may make a difference at the entry level, but past performance and attitude are what count. The committee members presented their recommendations to the chairman, who made the final selection of applicants.

After the selection has been made, the new leader experiences a period of transition and growth. Guiding, trusting, and allowing new leaders to take risks, make decisions, and grow from their accomplishments and mistakes are some of the most rewarding aspects of management. But it is certainly not a painless process for the newly appointed leader.

Reality shock[4] is a popular phrase used today to describe the transition from nursing student to new graduate. The following graphically describes the transition of a staff nurse to a leadership position. The staff may reject the new leader, peers may be jealous, and physicians may tease by saying: "I see you're one of them now. What we need is a nurse at the bedside, not another one wandering around with a clipboard doing nothing." The managerial sacrifices, commitment, and long hours are not always visible and understood. The ability to cope with personal feelings at this time is of prime concern.

Even when staff members express a desire for a new leader, the leader can expect to suffer periods of testing and challenge. For example, the units had long expressed a desire for on-the-spot supervision and support on all three shifts, 7 days a week. However, on selection of both evening and night clinical leaders and team leaders, a long and difficult period of adjustment followed this change in the organization. Even now, when leaders are replaced or new staff members are oriented, we see the "chicken coop theory" in action; that is, a new hen in the henhouse reduces egg production by 50%! It is a natural phenomenon that needs to be accepted and discussed before, during, and after it has been experienced. A new leader must avoid personalizing this natural reaction to the disequilibrium that occurs with change. If the reaction persists or if there is conflict, bring it out in the open—there is nothing like a thunderstorm to clear the air.

Use of personnel. Once you have written what you believe (philosophy), where you want to go (goals and objectives), how you are going to accomplish it (organizational chart), what each role is (job descriptions), and the kind of leaders required (selection of key people), the next step is to decide how many and what kind of persons are needed to attain your goals (use of personnel).

Decisions regarding use of personnel require an objectivity that can only be acquired through sharing ideas and needs. Ideally, a sense of shared purpose will develop within the decision-making body, promoting group interaction rather than reaction. For example, each unit had its own ideas, as well as policies, regarding staffing, hiring, and floating, because each unit had functioned independently prior to the chairman's arrival. As unit leaders looked at new ideas from a service rather than a unit point of view, it became increasingly easy to openly share both good and bad experiences, consider other options, take a risk, and initiate trial periods for new hiring and staffing policies. During this period, we learned that some things work and some things do not.

One of the things that worked was to have unit leaders or assistant chairmen continue to interview and hire new personnel for their respective units. They learned never to hire a problem. It is far better to be short of staff than to hire incompetent or difficult applicants just to fill positions. They also recognized that it is unfair to simply transfer a problem employee to another service. For example, if someone has a poor attendance record in one job, it is not likely to change in the next.

One of the things that did not work was continually floating staff between units, according to the changing needs of the service. Few staff members enjoy floating. Many even resent it for any number of reasons; either they feel the unit from which they were floated is busier, or that floats are given heavier assignments than the regular staff, or simply that they do not know where things are in the strange unit. The staff prompted the leadership group to look at the floating issue by collecting data illustrating the obvious inequities of the system. In this instance, budgeted positions were reallocated, and float books were used to record the frequency and name of individual nurses floated in each unit. These solutions were designed to prevent the problem from happening again. Many times the best solution to problems comes from the persons experiencing them. It does not take a lot of intelligence to simply gripe or agree; remember the best employee is the one who can suggest solutions.

Cost-effectiveness is a staggering responsibility for every manager, and effective use of personnel is a prime factor for consideration. Critical-care units are expensive. In this example, it was found that 30% of the registered nurses (RNs) in the hospital were assigned to specialty and critical-care units, caring for 10% of the total population.[5] The ratio of professional to nonprofessional nursing staff and the amount of nonnursing activities performed by RNs was examined. The result was a reduction in the number of RNs, with the subsequent hiring of nursing assistants and travel escorts to relieve nurses of some of the nonnursing duties such as setting up postoperative units or helping to transport recovery room patients to their rooms. Reallocation of budgeted money to clinical administration made it possible to have evening, night, and weekend secretarial coverage in all units. The impact of these changes was not only cost-effective, but it offered satisfying roles to non-professionals, increased efficiency, and removed frustrating, nonnursing duties from the nurse, freeing her for direct patient care.

Use of space. A very important, but all too often overlooked, aspect of ICUs is space. Space is needed for the endless and ever-increasing amounts of supplies and equipment in this technologically rich health care age, but space must also be provided for people. Relatives need a quiet, private place to wait, particularly in times of acute stress or for private conferences with physicians. Nursing staff members need a place for reports, teaching sessions, and private conferences, as well as a place to sit down quietly after an emotionally draining situation, or for a quick coffee break. Nursing leaders need space to complete necessary administrative paperwork and to hold private counseling sessions and interviews.

Storage areas, offices, conference rooms, and lounges may sound like luxury items to some, but the frustration level of people who work in high-pressure areas such as critical care can only be lowered by providing enough space for physical and psychological maneuverability. Overcrowding fosters aggression and dissatisfaction. Environment is a potent determinant of behavior and psychological well-being.

Communication

The need for interpersonal communication is so universal that it is often taken for granted. Communication does not just happen in an organization and there can never be enough. Informal or casual relationships are poor substitutes for formal communication channels.

Written communication. Unless information is written, many people will be missed in relaying information. Written policies and procedures are essential to an effective organization. Written documentation is the watchword of all quality assurance programs. Nursing histories and assessments, care plans, progress notes, and transfer and discharge notes are necessary to improve patient care and maintain standards of care. This need for written documentation must be reinforced by periodic nursing audits. Visitor brochures, critical-care flow sheets, and a service-oriented newsletter were developed in response to perceived needs for improved written communication within the area.

A daily report is written in each unit on all three shifts by the nurse in charge. One copy of the report remains in the unit, and one is forwarded to the director of nursing. Consequently information about patients and the general tone of the unit and individual views are expressed freely and shared daily with the director of nursing, thus keeping her in touch with all nursing areas in the department. This ongoing communication gives the staff a feeling of rapport with the director. The charge nurse also has the opportunity to deliver the report each morning and speak directly with the director.

Ad hoc reports to the director are written by the chairman as needed, concerning specific problems or issues faced by an area. Recommendations are included for consideration and/or action. These reports always receive prompt, direct, honest, and fair attention.

Annual reports are prepared for the director by each unit head nurse and staff. This is a valuable assessment tool, since it is often difficult to note changes and accomplishments on a day-to-day basis. These reports give everyone the opportunity to review the past year's progress and to set new goals for the upcoming year.

Writing is easier for some people than it is for others. Only if the staff recognizes the value of written communication will spontaneous and meaningful reports be forthcoming.

Regularly scheduled meetings. Regularly scheduled meetings with minutes distributed to appropriate groups will help open communication channels and facilitate understanding. It is better to have a short, informational meeting once a week than to have a long, heated discussion once a month prompted by a problem or crisis.

The nursing leadership group meets weekly and is led by the chairman. Leadership groups for each unit meet biweekly and are led by the assistant chairman responsible for the individual unit. Regular biweekly staff meetings are chaired by the charge nurse of the unit. Agendas vary according to needs; minutes are kept and posted. Various individuals such as medical directors, clinical pharmacists, psychiatric clinicians, unit coordinators, or chairmen of nursing committees are invited regularly to meetings to share information and participate in discussion or problem-solving sessions.

It was difficult at first for some leaders to convene and conduct meetings, but once the value of meetings was established, this problem diminished significantly. Now the regularly scheduled meetings are held regardless of how busy the units are at the time.

Committees. Committees are often the subject of jokes in management circles because to some leaders, committees are synonymous with ineffectiveness and red tape. Committees without purpose should be disbanded at once. Only if there are definite goals to be attained should a committee be continued.

Various committees have been invaluable. One is the advisory committee, which is a liaison group composed of staff representatives to the chairman. Matters of mutual interest and concern are discussed at the monthly meetings. The staff nurse who is the chairman of this committee also serves as the ICNS representative to the advisory committee to the director of nursing. Thus, information, questions, and recommendations can be brought directly from the staff to the director for consideration.

The medication incident review committee identifies early trends that may become problems. Appropriate policies, procedures, and practices are examined before the trends become serious issues.

Most leaders get their ideas from their people, and a committee is a good means of generating ideas. Also, a committee's interest and involvement in helping to solve problems will lessen the work load.

Staff development

Orientation and continuing education. Selecting and hiring personnel is only the first step in the development of a unit staff. Orientation, continuing education, and systematic, shared evaluations must follow. During the initial interview, we ask for a minimum commitment to the unit of 1 year, since it takes 3 to 6 months for new personnel to function at maximum effectiveness.

Stability of the nursing staff is a goal of any nursing unit. It is sometimes suggested that nurses be rotated regularly from one ICU to another to help them become experienced in a variety of specialities, thereby strengthening all units. It is not wise to force a regular rotation of nursing staff. If some nurses wish to work in another unit for a period of time, every effort should be made for them to do so. For example, each staff nurse in the postanesthesia recovery room rotated for 1 week to an acute care unit to become familiar with the care of a variety of critically ill patients. The staff viewed this experience as a satisfying learning opportunity. At the same time, a bond developed between the two unit staffs.

As a rule, the orientation and supervision needed to constantly bring each new rotation of nurses to a high level of performance in various units would be unwarranted. This practice is not satisfying to the individual nurse, it cannot promise a consistently high level of care, and it is not cost-effective.

In larger settings, it is advantageous to have an educational branch in the unit to provide orientation and continuing education of the staff. A brand new unit with every conceivable piece of equipment and an unlimited budget will not function well without an excellent nursing staff.

Evaluations. All nursing personnel should receive evaluations based on established expectations for performance. These evaluations should be given at 3 months, 6 months, and on the first anniversary of employment. Thereafter, an annual evaluation is sufficient unless a problem arises. Staff members need and want honest feedback on both their strengths and weaknesses to help them grow in their positions. Be truthful, but always be kind. They need loving critics, not just critics.

Some leaders tend to be lenient in evaluating staff members because they do not want to be the bad guy or disliked. A leader should never view evaluations as a popularity contest or simply mothering. Honest evaluation and subsequent development of personnel must go hand in hand with the organization of a service to achieve excellence in patient care.

WHAT TO DO WHEN IT DOESN'T WORK
Problem solving

When taking on the managerial role, you probably knew you could do the job and that you were exactly the right person for it. Perhaps you felt that given the chance, you could take care of problems you had identified and make the area an even better place to work.

Once in the job, however, many people find the glory of the job overshadowed by distressing realities. Never had one been exposed to so much criticism for decisions made and actions taken. It is vividly clear that change does not come easily or quickly and that others must be won over to really make change occur. Doubts often crowd in, and one wonders if some basic principle or some magic technique that would remove the conflicts is not missing. Managing conflict seems to be a large part of the job; and that had really not been bargained for.

The most important thing a manager can realize is that conflict is part of the role and that there will always be problems to solve. Some of these problems you can help solve, others will always seem to linger or recur, and new problems that were not anticipated will appear.

However, there is a definite approach to problem solving: do not become defensive, and do not put others on the defensive. It only adds an additional problem to be overcome. Defensiveness or the bulldozing approach (do as I say or get out) do not usually work and only serve as a barrier to communication.

Try to separate fact from emotion; do not take every criticism as a personal failure. Try to listen to what is being said. Get more than one opinion and look at all sides of an issue. Get those involved in the problem or conflict together. Tell them their help is needed for a good solution. Let everyone talk it out. Listen to the comments! Openness allows personnel to freely express their feelings and become less angry.

If necessary, document the problem with hard facts to prove a point. Gut feelings may prove to be correct, but no one should add positions, cut beds, change a long-used hospital procedure, or even terminate an employee without documentation. Provide proof that another course of action would be more consistent with organizational goals.

A manager should share problems with someone who can help. The effective problem solver must be realistic about the scope of the problem as well as the managerial skills required to solve it. Consider the following example of a problem-solving approach.

A supervisor making morning rounds in a twelve-bed surgical critical-care unit was confronted by a staff member who said, "What is the problem here? The morale has never been so low. No one seems motivated. We are already short-staffed, and a lot of people are going to leave if things don't change."

Feeling startled and hurt and somehow responsible for this situation, she talked with others and heard the following comments: "The time is terrible here." "I'm working a lot of overtime and no one cares." "This place is a pit!"

If new to the job, her first reaction might have been defensiveness and rationalization. After all, she was doing everything possible to help and hire more staff, but the staff just did not seem responsible and committed in hard times. However, she had learned from experience that defensiveness is easily conveyed to the staff, provoking anger and creating a wall between staff and management. Defensiveness prevents the group from taking an honest look at its problems in an attempt to change the situation. The supervisor had come to realize that her defensive rationalizations were not accurate and did not really make her feel any better.

The supervisor therefore approached the problem with the staff at their next meeting describing exactly how it had surfaced and what some of the staff members had said. A call for other comments about what the issues were and what might solve the problem prompted staff members to talk. It became apparent that they were tired and discouraged not only about short-staffing, but also about patients in the unit. The unit was normally a very acute unit with rapid patient turnover. The staff thrived in this type of atmosphere. For the past 5 weeks, seven patients had remained in the twelve-bed unit because of the severity of their illness and complications. Consequently, the patient turnover in the other five beds was so rapid that acutely ill surgical patients often did not have a chance for a reasonable stay because room had to be made for other critically ill patients from surgery.

This action-oriented staff felt they were getting nowhere with the seven chronic patients, several of whom would probably die, and that they were cheating others who could profit from their care. Neither physicians nor the administration seemed to care about the situation. The surgical schedule forged ahead at any cost. The following actions were taken as a result of the staff meeting:

1. The supervisor spoke with the unit's medical director about the feelings expressed by the staff and requested help. A meeting was planned between the medical director, chief surgical resident, and nursing staff to discuss the chronic patients, their progress, and future plans.

2. The supervisor began to closely document overtime, absenteeism, the rapidity of discharge from the unit, and the number of patients returned to the unit after discharge. It became obvious that everyone was overworked and that some patients were leaving too soon. There were too many sick patients and not enough beds to accommodate them, since approximately 60% of the beds were never vacated.

3. The supervisor presented these findings to the head of the service, director of nursing, and medical director.

Although the decision that had to be made was a difficult one, everyone felt the situation would become worse if ignored. The following decisions were made: chronic patients were moved to other areas as soon as possible to open up beds for acute patients, the surgical schedule was reduced slightly in volume, and the unit patient census was temporarily decreased from twelve to ten to ensure adequate nurse/patient ratios without excessive overtime during this period of low staffing.

The situation was alleviated over the next 2 months. Physicians occasionally asked that the census go to eleven or twelve patients for 24 hours to accommodate emergency cases. During this time the nursing staff willingly worked overtime to provide coverage and adopted the philosophy to safely provide quality care for as many patients as possible. As new staff members were hired and oriented, the census returned to twelve. If the problem had been ignored as a hot issue about which nothing could be done, the staff would have become increasingly discouraged and demoralized, thus perpetuating the problem.

An important point to note about this situation is that the solution to the problem was not pleasing to everyone. Although the surgeons went along with the decreased census, they were angry and blamed the nursing staff for allowing a low-staffing situation to occur. The nursing staff, on the other hand, felt the physicians had not been making appropriate decisions regarding placement of chronic patients and had unrealistically pushed the surgical schedule. Discussion on these issues recurred over the next several months. Thus, the period of problem resolution often continues to be stressful.

Problems would be a lot simpler if only clearly defined issues had to be dealt with; the fact is that most of the time there is no absolute right or wrong. Solutions to problems that are fair and supportive of the people within the organization, as well as of benefit to organizational objectives, should be sought.

Motivation

Do any of these phrases sound familiar?

Nobody loves me and I don't love anybody.
I am going to be an old maid.
I have lived my best years and I'm on my way downhill.
Christmas is only for children.
My (head nurse or supervisor) is picky. I think she really has a grudge against
   me.
I'm always tired no matter how much sleep I get.
My roommate is getting grumpy. I wonder what's wrong with her.
Life is dull. Color it gray.
Here I am ____ years old and I have not accomplished a thing. I run around
   the unit all day and nobody appreciates me.
I'm not getting anywhere.
I'm going to quit this job. Life wasn't meant to be wasted.
What's the use. Ugh!

Just about everyone can identify with some of these feelings. If you are in a management position, you probably have seen many staff members exhibit them. The difficult question is how to treat these feelings. What role can a manager take to help someone become less pessimistic and more constructively involved in work and in the unit?

There are innumerable theories of motivation. Although the structure of each is different, one basic thread is common to all. Everyone needs to feel needed and worthwhile as an individual. Individuals need to feel good about themselves.

From the time you begin to work with a group as a manager, give personnel credit for what they do. Often this is something that has to be a conscious effort. Many are quick to praise a staff member who has written several new procedures or developed classes for ongoing education or done something else beyond the expectations for the average staff nurse. However, credit needs to be given for little things that are so often overlooked. Consistently thank the staff for their team support with overtime when the unit is busy or tell a staff nurse that she has done a nice job with a sick patient or a heavy assignment. Try to focus on the best in people: a sense of humor, an ability to look objectively at both sides of a problem, or an ability to work well with others as a dependable team member. If the only comments staff members hear are constructive criticisms, they may minimize their contacts with leadership, thus decreasing communication, motivation, and purpose.

The staff especially needs your support in conflict. Gather all the facts from both sides before making a decision concerning the staff—remain neutral! Never allow your actions to cause an individual to lose face in front of the group. The manager's role is to be a mediator in the conflict, a synthesizer of the facts, and a catalyst in developing a solution.

If you feel that a staff nurse or another leader for whom you are responsible should have approached a problem differently, take the person aside and review the issues and better ways of handling them. Your goal is staff development, not undermining feelings of self-worth. Staff members who are helped to grow in their work will be more eager to take risks and try new skills, such as more difficult patient assignments or charge duties. They know they will learn from these experiences. Constant correction with little reward will discourage staff involvement.

Start small in developing the staff. Give the staff assignments that are manageable and can be completed in a reasonable period of time. For instance, asking one staff member to revise an outdated procedure manual or develop one from scratch is unrealistic. The person may be eager to attempt it, but will soon discover that it is a long and overwhelming task. However, if several members assume the responsibility, each revising one or two procedures, they can easily complete the task and feel a sense of accomplishment. A unit committee should review the completed procedures for similarity of style and format. The manual can then be presented for administrative review and approval.

Whether writing goals, objectives, standards of care, or procedures, encourage staff members to be practical. In this way their efforts will have impact in the area. Clear, practical standards are better understood, believed in, and used. To compose lengthy dissertations that can never be implemented is a waste of valuable time.

Approach staff members with the philosophy that they deserve and are expected to develop to their fullest potential. Give them the opportunity to grow and assume new skills. Assign tasks that give increased responsibility. Have staff nurses assigned to work regularly with orientees as the orientees begin work in the unit or move to an off shift. As staff nurses become competent and organized in the delivery of patient care, orient them to charge duties with the head nurse even if permanent charge people are used. As head nurse, assign other senior staff persons to run a staff meeting when you are away. As a supervisor, if you interview personnel, have head nurses interview with you occasionally. Share your ideas and thoughts with them. Let them know why you approach a situation as you do.

Build your leaders to replace you. Constantly communicate with them about your goals and have them help with problems so that they can expand their understanding of your role and their ability to cope with broader concepts of the organization. Your leaders, whether supervisors, head nurses, or strong senior staff nurses, are the key support in your staff. As they gain management and leadership ability, they will also begin to work with and develop other members of the staff, thereby strengthening the organization.

Recognize that some people can never be helped or motivated. You are running an organization, not a social service department. In every area, there are three groups of people. A small percentage are self-starters who enjoy their work and the challenge of change. A small percentage are magnets for negativity. Nothing ever seems right for them. They are chronically malcontent with work. The majority of people have their ups and downs. This third group can be developed as energetic supporters of the area's goals.

There will be times when individual staff members reevaluate their personal status and wonder where they are going. When they are doubtful and uncertain, diffuse complaining and dwelling on negatives can rapidly spread among staff and decrease morale. Keep lines of communication open with the staff. Be sensitive to changes in mood. Constructively work on problems in the unit and realize that staff members play an important part in their own morale and the morale of their peers.

As for the manager, be positive! Optimism is an important attitudinal characteristic of a manager. You set the tone for the staff in your area. If you feel that things are hopeless and nothing will change, this idea will be conveyed to your people. Effective leaders attract support and enthusiasm because they are positive, purposeful, and believe in what they are doing. People want to be a part of that kind of an organization.

WHERE IT CAN TAKE YOU

Do not expect change and staff development to occur overnight; it will take time. If you are new in your role, it will take at least a year to know your people, develop them, establish the goals and framework of your area, and feel comfortable in your role. In succeeding years, the framework will become more solid and you will effectively set long-range goals.

As staff members develop, they will be better able to cope with the day-to-day operation of their units. As lower-level management personnel assume responsibility for crisis intervention and problem solving, you will be able to set goals focusing on the design of innovative approaches to patient care and staff development. For instance, one established intensive care nursing service developed the following types of educational programs:

1. A refined orientation program for new staff with established objectives, teaching outlines, and audiovisual aids for each content area
2. An advanced critical-care course for senior staff in the area
3. Management seminars for leaders in the area
4. Acute care conferences within the hospital
5. Community and national teaching conferences

Realistically, there will be moments when you wish you could throw the problems, conflicts, failures, and losses in the wastebasket and walk away. But continually strengthening team efforts, leaders growing in their ability to manage, and improved quality of caring for patients and their families make you know you are part of an effective organization.

REFERENCES

1. Beasley, N.: Main street merchant, Whittlesey House, New York, 1948, McGraw-Hill Book Co., p. 61.
2. Philosophy, the intensive care nursing service, Department of Nursing, Massachusetts General Hospital, Boston.
3. Objectives of the intensive care nursing service, Department of Nursing, Massachusetts General Hospital, Boston.
4. Kramer, M.: Reality shock: why nurses leave nursing, St. Louis, 1974, The C. V. Mosby Co.
5. 1975 Annual Report Statistics of the Intensive Care Nursing Service, Department of Nursing, Massachusetts General Hospital, Boston.

CONSIDERATIONS FOR PATIENT CARE

In Chapter 12 William C. Shoemaker provides a guide to monitoring in critical-care units. From the easily obtained, most frequently used vital signs to the more complex modalities, he tells why the parameter is monitored and identifies the normal ranges and ramifications of derangements.

Frequently, prospective critical-care nurses are intimidated by the lights, alarms, and lines associated with monitoring. Physicians and nurses new to a particular unit often find that they must acquire new skills to operate equipment that is unfamiliar to them. However, only the techniques differ. The basic principles of biomedical electronic equipment are the same, even though the knobs and buttons are in different places.

Perhaps the most difficult aspect of complex forms of monitoring is the ability of the nurse and physician to remember the patient as a person. Too often we lapse into the cadence of technology and neglect the fears and feelings of the person we are working so hard to help. It is exceedingly rude to carry on personal conversations within hearing of the patient. The time would be better spent with the patient, comforting, listening, or talking of things to which the patient could relate. Even the critically ill derive comfort from a touch, a glance, and a gentle word. It is exasperating to hear nurses and physicians refer to bed 6 or the lady with the ruptured spleen. It is safe to assume that these health workers have never been on the receiving end, a consumer of critical-care services.

So long as we bear in mind that increasingly sophisticated technology enables us to provide better care for sicker patients, monitoring can be kept in perspective. Only when we lose sight of our goal does monitoring become an end in itself.

Dennis M. Greenbaum (Chapter 13) succinctly describes a data collection system that is simple, expedient, and useful. Statistical data are invaluable in determining needs for equipment, staff, space, and programs. A projected budget should take into consideration the type of data outlined by Green-baum; using the same figures for several years will reveal seasonal trends. Such information can be used in planning vacation schedules and recruiting campaigns.

Communication, a challenge in any organization, becomes increasingly essential when stress and anxiety are factors to be considered. The publication of actual facts and figures prevents staff members from exaggerating trends in mortality and morbidity.

In addition to the patient statistics mentioned, a newsletter might contain other information of interest to all members of the unit staff such as notes on new employees, engagements, weddings, and pregnancies. News of planned staffing changes, equipment purchases, and other information is better delivered accurately in the news publication than by rumor. Minimal effort is needed to produce nonstatistical portions of the communication. Notes kept by the responsible party can be typed and copied in a short time.

For nursing staff and between-shift communication, a message book is invaluable. A simple 8½- by 11-inch spiral binder kept readily available at the nurses' station encourages staff members to make entries. One pitfall is the tendency for sarcasm in messages, but it can be handled without too much difficulty.

When designing newsletters it is wise to incorporate pertinent information from areas other than the unit and make the publication available to them. Every effort should be made to minimize the atmosphere of elitism, estrangement, and alienation between the critical-care units and general areas of the hospital.

Neil M. Goodwin (Chapter 14) provides an opportunity to share a critical-care world that few of us will ever experience. Despite all sorts of incredible diseases, complications, and obstacles, his South African team is able to use available resources to the maximum. He has developed a team that not only crosses specialty lines, but cultural, religious, and historical barriers. The witch doctor, herbalist, and the patient's family and tribe are all part of the team working toward the patient's recovery. Goodwin graphically shows how important the psychosocial aspects of illness really are. We so often forget to take into consideration the patient's background, particularly during the recovery period. We care little that the patient may never have eaten potatoes, salad, and white bread; generally, if it is on the menu, that is what we serve. In South Africa, there is more respect for the individuality of patients. A great deal can be learned from our colleagues in less fortunate areas, and Goodwin gives us a glimpse of another world.

CHAPTER 12

Monitoring the critically ill patient

William C. Shoemaker

> Science is measurement.
>
> *Helmholtz*

Provisions for monitoring functions are a necessary part of planning a new ICU or remodeling an existing ICU. Careful assessment of expected patient needs, as well as human resources, may prevent wasteful expenditures for inappropriate monitoring systems. Equally wasteful are facilities that inadequately meet patient needs, JCAH standards, and expectations of referring physicians; under these circumstances the facilities must be redeveloped to meet the real needs. The present state of the art allows for a wide variety of approaches to patient monitoring, but decisions regarding the commercially available systems to use depend largely on the overall purposes, which in turn depend on the clinical load of the hospital, referral patterns, and available expertise in critical care.

Usually the ICU should have 5% to 10% of acute care beds in the community hospital; the number will be two or three times this figure in teaching hospitals and referral centers (trauma and burn centers, cancer centers, and other tertiary care centers). Although the extent and sophistication of physiological monitoring has been more advanced in the universities and referral centers, many community hospitals have already achieved these levels or are not far behind.

The single most important factor in the choice of monitoring facilities is the commitment of the administration, medical staff, and nursing service. Deficiencies of the physical plant and human resources may limit ICU function, but they may be corrected (at some cost); expertise, if not available, may be recruited. However, inertia of the administration or staff reluctance may produce an insoluble impasse.

The monitoring functions of an ICU vary from simple electrocardiographic (ECG) surveillance to sophisticated cardiorespiratory functions. The type, extent, and complexity of monitoring functions will depend on the overall purpose and function of the ICU. For example, the cardiac ICU and postanesthesia recovery room may only require continuous display of the ECG, heart rate, arterial pressure, and venous pressure at the bedside. In addition to these, the surgical and multidisciplinary ICU may require facilities for advanced cardiorespiratory monitoring with the Swan-Ganz thermodilution cardiac output catheter, arterial and mixed venous blood gases, blood volume, serum electrolytes, and osmolarity. The respiratory ICU may have a sophisticated mass spectrometer for continuous monitoring of expired gases, end-tidal CO_2, dead space, oxygen consumption ($\dot{V}O_2$), and CO_2 production ($\dot{V}CO_2$). This chapter briefly summarizes the state of the art for the most commonly used monitoring systems that are applicable for the surgical and multidisciplinary ICU.

No single aspect of the care of the critically ill patient is more essential to survival than the prompt recognition of life-threatening problems and expeditious correction of these deficiencies. However, it is often difficult to determine the amount or rate of administration and type of therapy that is most efficient in achieving this end. Inaccurate physiological evaluation of the ICU patient is likely to jeopardize survival by inviting inappropriate and ineffectual therapy.

A dozen or more important physiological variables are commonly used to monitor ICU patients. These variables range from routine, vital signs to complex, hemodynamic and oxygen transport variables. They are listed here in approximate order of frequency of use, beginning with the most frequently monitored:

1. Arterial blood pressure
2. Heart rate
3. Temperature
4. Hematocrit and hemoglobin concentration
5. Central venous pressure (CVP)
6. Urine output rate and specific gravity
7. Electrocardiogram (ECG)
8. Serum electrolytes and blood chemistries
9. Arterial blood gases (ABG) and pH
10. Blood volume
11. Plasma and urine osmolality, osmolar and free-water clearances
12. Electroencephalogram (EEG)
13. Intracranial pressures
14. Pulmonary arterial and precapillary wedge pressures
15. Cardiac output and hemodynamic variables
16. O_2 transport variables; O_2 availability, O_2 consumption ($\dot{V}O_2$), and O_2 extraction rate

The order of frequency of use is the opposite of their physiological specificity and significance; that is, commonly used variables are good for screening but are nonspecific. The more complex physiological measurements often give specific and quantitative information needed to restore circulation and provide the best chance for survival.[1]

ARTERIAL PRESSURE

Arterial pressures and heart rate, the so-called vital signs, are the most commonly used monitoring variables. They are part of routine admission notes, physical examinations, daily nursing care, and standard screening for all acutely ill patients. Vital signs should be taken and recorded at intervals to provide a running graphic account. Normal arterial blood pressures (BP) are usually given as 120/80 mm Hg for healthy young adults, but may be as low as 90/60 in young adults. BP increases gradually with age. The upper limit of normal for systolic pressures is 100 plus the patient's age; systolic pressures over 160 and diastolic pressures over 90 mm Hg are usually considered hypertensive. It is important to know the patient's normal pressures to avoid giving vasopressors unnecessarily to maintain pressure of 120/80 mm Hg or to withhold therapy in the previously hypertensive patient whose postoperative values are 120/80 mm Hg.

Pulse pressure, which is the difference between systolic and diastolic pressures, is more informative. Decreased pulse pressure often precedes the fall in diastolic pressure in the patient who is developing hypovolemic shock, and widening of the pulse pressure occurs with restoration of volume.

Intra-arterial pressure measurements

Continuous recording of pressures that are more accurate than cuff pressure may be obtained by a system of intra-arterial catheters, pressure transducers, and a recording apparatus. They are indicated in patients with shock, critical illness, unstable BP, intraoperative and postoperative monitoring of high-risk patients, patients with marked peripheral vasoconstriction, and those needing frequent arterial blood gas (ABG) analyses. The common sites for arterial catheters include radial, femoral, and axillary arteries; the latter is preferred.[2]

Arterial pressures taken with the cuff are often inaccurate. On the average, intra-arterial pressures are usually 5 to 30 mm Hg higher than cuff pressure measurements. Early in the patient's hospital stay, pressures should be taken in both arms, because unilateral arteriosclerotic or traumatic vascular lesions may produce differences between the left and right sides. In vascular trauma, cuff pressures of the arms may differ from each other and with the legs. Usually femoral pressures average 5 to 10 mm Hg higher than brachial pressures.

Arterial pressures decrease with shock, but usually the fall in arterial pressure occurs after protective compensations are exhausted and may take a considerable period of time after the hemorrhage has occurred. We have observed severely reduced cardiac output for 40 minutes to 2 hours before reduction in arterial pressures. Intra-arterial pressure monitoring is mandatory for optimal therapy in critical illness.

HEART RATE

Tachycardia, which is defined as heart rates over 100 beats/min, is also a nonspecific cardiorespiratory variable. Its increase suggests blood flow and blood volume deficits; the faster the heart rate, the greater the hypovolemia or cardiac impairment. Tachycardias associated with cardiac problems are termed *dysrhythmias* and require ECG and other measures for specific diagnosis. Increased heart rates occur with infections, anxiety, stress, fever, exercise, pain, discomfiture, etc. With irregularities of the cardiac rhythm, apical as well as radial rates should be compared. A slow pulse rate or bradycardia in the face of low cardiac output is an ominous sign suggesting inadequate coronary blood flow.

TEMPERATURE

Rectal temperature is taken routinely in ill patients to indicate possible sepsis. It may be taken orally when significant elevations are not expected. Skin temperatures have been used to assess peripheral blood flow; large differences between rectal and big toe temperatures suggest reduced peripheral flow, and increases in toe temperature with narrowing of the temperature gradients suggest improved flow.

HEMATOCRIT

Hematocrit is a measure of the percentage of red cells in a sample of venous blood. It has been widely used for assessment of blood loss after trauma and surgery; decreased hematocrit values are seen after hemorrhage. The decrease does not represent a direct effect of blood loss per se, but rather an indirect compensatory effect from transcapillary refilling of the plasma volume by extracellular fluid. The hematocrit fall, therefore, is a measure of a compensatory reaction, not a direct measure of blood loss. Hemoglobin concentrations, which are about one third the numerical value of hematocrit values, may be used instead of the latter.

It takes time for this compensation to occur. If a patient exsanguinates rapidly, the first and last drop of blood will have nearly the same hematocrit. Blood loss of 500 ml is replaced by interstitial water initially at about 1 ml/min for the first few hours and then at successively decreasing rates over an 18-hour period.[3] In severe hemorrhage, replacement occurs at two or three times this rate.[4] Therefore, it is useful to measure serial hematocrits at about 4-hour intervals in patients with suspected bleeding.

Serial hematocrits may be useful in the early period of postoperative and traumatic shock when covert blood loss is suspected. When patients are given large volumes of fluids, especially colloids, as well as multiple transfusions, the changes in hematocrit cannot be interpreted as reflecting blood volumes; that is, hematocrit values of ICU patients are not correlated with blood volume measurements.[5]

Since the hematocrit is a static measurement of red cell concentration, it is affected by either gains or losses of plasma water, as well as gains or losses of red cells. Indeed, all four shifts may be occurring at the same time: fluids administered intravenously, fluids leaking from the plasma to the interstitial space, red cells being transfused, whereas other red cells form microthrombi and drop out of the circulation. Under these conditions, small changes in hematocrit are difficult to interpret accurately. Although hematocrits may be a good screening test for gross changes in patients with hemorrhage, it is not a reliable estimation of blood volume.

CENTRAL VENOUS PRESSURE (CVP)

Because of its simplicity and availability, CVP monitoring is often routinely used to guide fluid therapy in trauma and emergency conditions in which facilities for rapid blood volume measurements are not available.[6,7] The catheters are simple to place, and the pressure values are easy to read. The normal values are −2 (on inspiration) to +4 (on expiration) cm water. However, a healthy ambulatory person who is lying down may have CVP values averaging 5 cm water, but gradually the CVP decreases as the vascular tree accommodates. Unfortunately, many factors may influence CVP: cardiac performance; blood volume; vascular tone; administration of vasopressors; and intrathoracic pressure changes from hydrothorax, pneumothorax, pulmonary emboli, mechanical ventilation, ascites, and chronic obstructive lung disease. Therefore CVP is not an index of any single function but a reflection of various combinations of many influences. There was no correlation between CVP and blood volume values in a large group of ICU patients.[5] Nevertheless, it is generally accepted that if a patient has a CVP greater than 15 cm water, heart failure or fluid overload is present, and fluid administration should be curtailed. However, we have seen improvement in myocardial performance of postoperative patients with high CVP, both with and without significant blood volume deficits, after the expansion of their blood volumes.[5] When CVP values exceed 15, a Swan-Ganz balloon catheter should be used to obtain precapillary wedge pressures.

URINE OUTPUT RATE

The hourly urine output rate obtained with an indwelling urethral catheter is an estimate of renal perfusion, provided there is an adequate blood volume and the patient did not have preexisting renal disease.[7] Urine output is easy to measure and involves only minimal expense; however, it is not foolproof. The most common cause of oliguria or anuria is a plugged catheter. Irrigation (using aseptic precautions) at regular intervals is essential to ensure accuracy of measurements. Urinary specific gravity may be used as a screening test of the concentrating capacity of the kidney.

In resuscitation from acute injury, hemorrhage, and postoperative states, decreased urine flow may reflect low blood volume, poor perfusion of the kidney, or the onset of acute renal failure.[7]

ELECTROCARDIOGRAPHIC (ECG) MONITORING

The ECG pattern is one of the most frequently used devices for continuous electronic monitoring of the acutely ill patient over long periods of time. The ECG is essential for acute myocardial infarction, dysrhythmias, and other electromechanical problems. ECG waveforms may be constantly displayed and recorded when desired on a permanent record at the patient's bedside, as well as at a central monitor station. This provides a continuous graphic display for early recognition of dysrhythmias and electromechanical changes.

ECG monitoring is also useful in the diagnosis of cardiac complications in the acutely injured patient, postoperative patient, and septic patient. Considering the small amount of useful information gained in these groups, ECG monitoring is probably overemphasized because these patients do not have a high incidence of significant dysrhythmias. In essence, ECG monitoring is specific for early diagnosis of dysrhythmias and electrical disturbances of the heart in acute cardiac conditions, but is not particulary useful in patients with noncardiac conditions. However, dysrhythmias may develop from inadequate oxygen delivery, hypovolemia, and hypoxemia.

SERUM ELECTROLYTES AND BLOOD CHEMISTRIES

In acute illness, accidents, and postoperative states, serum Na^+, K^+, Cl^-, Ca^{++}, Mg^{++}, $PO_4^=$, and HCO_3^- are routinely taken as are blood glucose, lactate, blood urea nitrogen (BUN), and creatinine values. Although these are biochemical tests used to establish or rule out various diagnoses, they are also used to monitor changes in rapidly developing acute illnesses. Of particular importance are dysrhythmias from hypokalemia associated with alkalosis and hyperkalemia associated with acidosis; hyperglycemia associated with diabetes, stress, trauma, and head injury; hypoglycemia associated with insulin reactions, insulinoma, nutritional deficiency; lactacidemia associated with low cardiac output, hypovolemia, cardiogenic shock; increasing BUN and creatinine associated with renal failure; low plasma Ca^{++} after multiple transfusions, pancreatitis, etc. Serial values of these variables are useful to follow the course of disease states and to assess the adequacy of therapy.

ARTERIAL BLOOD GASES (ABG) AND pH

ABG and pH are useful analyses to screen for pulmonary gas exchange (p. 181). Since the usefulness of ABG analyses has been demonstrated, they have rapidly gained popularity and are now used routinely in critically ill patients, especially those with suspected pulmonary complications. Although clinical judgment is adequate to assess many physiological variables, it is virtually impossible to guess what the blood gases or pH is likely to be in the acutely ill patient. It is mandatory, therefore, to make these measurements rather than rely on clinical impressions. Following are situations in which blood gases are indicated in the initial evaluation and workup:

1. Critically ill patients with tachypnea, dyspnea, acute respiratory distress syndrome (ARDS), or for patients with suspected respiratory problems
2. Patients who have sustained accidental trauma, extensive surgery, and other acute emergencies

---

NORMAL VALUES FOR ROOM AIR (FIO_2 0.21)

Arterial O_2 tension, PaO_2, 80 to 100 torr

Mixed venous O_2 tension, $P\bar{v}O_2$, 35 to 50 torr

Arterial O_2 saturation, SaO_2, 97%

Arterial O_2 content, CaO_2, 18-20 ml/100 ml

Mixed venous O_2 content, $C\bar{v}O_2$, 12-15 ml/100 ml

Arteriovenous O_2 difference, $a\bar{v}DO_2$, 4.6 ml/100 ml

Arterial CO_2 tension, $PaCO_2$, 36 to 44 torr

Mixed venous CO_2 tension, $P\bar{v}CO_2$, 40 to 46 torr

pH, 7.36 to 7.44

Bicarbonate, HCO_3^-, 25 to 28 mEq/L

Base excess or deficit, +3 to −3 mEq/L

---

3. Patients who are receiving controlled or assisted mechanical ventilation
4. Patients receiving oxygen therapy
5. Preoperative evaluation
6. Patients with fluid and electrolyte problems
7. Restlessness, anxiety, or mental confusion
8. Patients with drug overdose
9. Patients who fail to respond after administration of an anesthetic

BLOOD VOLUME

Nothing is as specific and definitive for estimating the volume of blood loss as an accurate and readily available measure of the volume of blood remaining.[7,10] Indications for blood volume measurements are suspected blood loss after accidental trauma, postoperative states, unstable vital signs, shock states, critically ill patients suspected of having blood volume deficits or excesses, dehydration or overhydration states, and patients whose marginal cardiovascular system requires careful titration of blood volume replacements. Over 50% of patients who were studied on entrance to a surgical ICU had blood volume deficits between 0.5 and 2.0 liters, and another 13% had blood volumes in excess of their predicted norms.[8]

PLASMA AND URINE OSMOLALITY, OSMOLAR AND FREE WATER CLEARANCES

Traditionally BUN and creatinine levels are used to diagnose acute renal failure (ARF), but renal function in the critically ill patient also may be assessed by routine monitoring of plasma (Posm) and urine (Uosm) osmolality, as well as osmolar and free water clearances.

Osmolality of body fluids is measured by the freezing point depression method (Fiske osmometer) or vapor pressure method. The $\frac{Uosm}{Posm}$ ratio can be easily calculated from these two measurements. If the rate of urinary output (UO) is also measured in the same specimen, the osmolar clearance (Cosm) is calculated as follows:

$$Cosm = \frac{Uosm}{Posm} \times UO$$

and free water clearance:

$$C_{H_2O} = UO - Cosm$$

The capacity of the kidney to concentrate urine is its most sensitive and important function. Although this is often inferred from urine output rates and specific gravity, the concentrating capacity is far better assessed by: (1) the ratio of urinary to plasma osmolalities, with ratios above 1.7 suggesting good concentrative ability; (2) osmolar clearances, expressing the rate of removal of solutes from the plasma; normally osmolar clearance is 120 ml/hr and is markedly decreased in ARF; and (3) free water clearance, which more explicitly takes into account the rate of urinary output and is an extremely sensitive indicator of the early onset of postoperative ARF. Normally free water clearance is strongly negative, such as -25 to -100 ml/hr, but values close to zero precede the development of ARF. For example, a patient with urine osmolality of 330, plasma osmolality of 300 mOsm/L, and urine output of 100 ml/hr has a relatively normal osmolar clearance (110 ml/hr), but the free water clearance of -10/hr indicates high output renal failure.[11]

ELECTROENCEPHALOGRAPHY (EEG)

EEG is frequently used as a diagnostic test in critically ill patients with a central nervous system (CNS) deficit. Serial EEG may be used to monitor changes in electrical activity in patients with a head injury and those who are semicomatose or comatose with progressively deteriorating comatose states. It is also used to evaluate the possibility of brain death. Continuous EEG monitoring is occasionally used in the administration of anesthetics and for surgery on the carotid arteries under certain critical conditions.

INTRACRANIAL PRESSURES

Continuous intracranial pressure measurements and recordings can be obtained by one of two methods: a hollow, fluid-filled Richmond screw[12] placed in the subdural space and a Scott cannula[12] placed in the lateral ventricle. Both transducers and catheters are inserted through small burr holes placed in the parietal region of the calvaria with a 1% or 2% lidocaine local anesthetic; the nondominant hemisphere is usually selected. The Richmond screw is attached to a pressure transducer and recording system for measurement, graphic display, and recording of intracranial pressures. Sampling and draining cerebrospinal fluid (CSF) through the screw is not possible.

In contrast, the Scott cannula is connected with a sterile closed fluid system, usually with stopcocks having resealable rubber part covers* that allow aspiration of CSF by a sterile needle when needed. The ventricular fluid may also be withdrawn for culture and chemical analyses. A sterile closed fluid system, which is attached to a pressure transducer and recording system, may be used for intermittent drainage of CSF during periods of intracranial hypertension and for direct display of the pressure waveforms or numerical readout.

PULMONARY ARTERIAL (PAP) AND PRECAPILLARY WEDGE (WP) PRESSURES

Pulmonary arterial pressures (systolic, diastolic, and mean) are routinely measured during diagnostic cardiac catheterization. With the introduction of the balloon-tipped, flow-directed (Swan-Ganz) catheter, pulmonary arterial pressures (PAP) and precapillary wedge pressures (WP) have been frequently used at the bedside of the ICU patient as a diagnostic aid to differentiate acute cardiac failure from fluid volume abnormalities and pulmonary problems.[13]

This catheter is extremely useful as a monitoring procedure to guide fluid therapy, particularly in patients with postoperative conditions, as well as myocardial infarction, or other types of cardiac problems. Indications for its use include shock and trauma states, critically ill patients whose fluid and circulatory status is in doubt, and patients with acute myocardial infarction.

In myocardial infarction, the expected hemodynamic pattern is hypotension, low cardiac output, increased ventricular filling pressure (wedge pressure), and usually decreased ventricular contractility and compliance. PAP and wedge pressure are useful ways to monitor progress of the disease and responses to various therapeutic interventions.

Complications of the Swan-Ganz catheter include pulmonary infarction, small pulonary emboli, rupture of small branches of the pulmonary artery, knotting, dysrhythmias, and infection.

CARDIAC OUTPUT AND HEMODYNAMIC VARIABLES

The most important aspects of the circulatory system are blood pressure, volume, flow, and oxygen transport. The first is easily measured and automated; the second takes more time and effort but is simple in concept and relatively straightforward technically. Measurement of blood flow is more complex and fraught with potential errors. The recent development of thermodilution balloon flotation catheters with computerized calculation has greatly simplified measurements, but has not entirely eliminated methodological errors.

---

*Pharmaseal Labs, Glendale, Calif. 91201.

Direct Fick technique

Fick postulated in 1887 that if the oxygen content of arterial (CaO_2) and mixed venous ($C\bar{v}O_2$) blood were known, as well as the O_2 consumption ($\dot{V}O_2$), then cardiac output (CO) could be calculated as follows:

$$CO = \frac{\dot{V}O_2}{CaO_2 - C\bar{v}O_2}$$

This requires measurement of $\dot{V}O_2$ by spirometry and simultaneous anaerobic sampling of blood from a systemic artery and the right ventricle or pulmonary artery at the same time. O_2 contents are measured either directly by manometry or by an electric O_2 consumption cell,* or they are calculated from hemoglobin concentrations and saturations by co-oximetry.† The direct Fick method for estimating cardiac output has become the standard against which other methods are evaluated.

Thermodilution method for measurement of cardiac output

The concept of thermal dilution is an application of the indicator dilution principle in which the indicator is a measured quantity of iced 5% glucose solution, and the dilution of solution into the flowing stream of blood is measured by a calibrated thermocouple, which is about 10 cm upstream from the point of injection. The advantages of thermodilution over those of the indicated dilution method with indocyanine green dye are that little or no recirculation of the thermal indicator occurs, and it may be repeated frequently. It does not require removal of blood for photometric analysis, and it may be used in conjunction with the blood floatation catheter to obtain simultaneous pulmonary arterial and wedge pressures.[13]

Calculation of hemodynamic variables

All volume and flow measurements can be indexed by dividing by the patient's body surface area to provide standardized or normalized hemodynamic values of patients with widely varying size. Furthermore, various derived hemodynamic variables may be calculated from pressure and flow data using standard formulas (Table 5); these include cardiac index, stroke index, left and right ventricular stroke work, left and right cardiac work, central blood volume, systemic (peripheral) vascular resistance, pulmonary vascular resistance, tension-time index, and mean systolic ejection rate.

OXYGEN TRANSPORT VARIABLES

Cardiac output, which is the rate of blood flow pumped by the heart, is one of the most important hemodynamic aspects of the circulation. But the essential metabolic function of circulation is bulk transport of gases (O_2 and CO_2),

---

*Lexington Instruments, Boston, Mass.
†Lexington Instruments Co-oximeter, Boston, Mass.

Table 5. Selected monitored variables: their units, formulas, and normal values

Abbreviation	Variable name	Unit	Formula	Normal values
MAP	Mean arterial pressure	mm Hg	(Systolic + 2 × diastolic) ÷ 3	80-98
CVP	Central venous pressure	cm H_2O	Direct measurement	0-10
Hg	Hemoglobin concentration	g/100 ml	Direct measurement	12-15
MPAP	Mean pulmonary arterial pressure	mm Hg	Direct measurement	10-18
WP	Pulmonary arterial wedge pressure	mm Hg	Direct measurement	2-12
BV def	Blood volume deficit or excess	Liter/M^2	Direct measurement	2.74 men
				2.37 women
CI	Cardiac index	Liter/min/M^2	Direct measurement	2.8-3.6
LVSW	Left ventricular stroke work	gM/M^2	LVSW = SI × MAP × .0144	44-68
LCW	Left cardiac work	kgM/M_2	LCW = CI × MAP × .0144	3-4.5
SVR	Systemic vascular resistance	dyne cm/sec^5M^2	SVR = 80 (MAP − CVP) ÷ CI	1800-2600
PVR	Pulmonary vascular resistance	dyne cm/sec^5M^2	PVR = 80 (MPAP − WP) ÷ CI	180-350
HR	Heart rate	beats/min	Direct measurement	65-80
Temp	Temperature	°F	Direct measurement	98-98.6
O_2 avail	O_2 availability	ml/min/M^2	O_2 avail = CI × Cao_2 × 10	500-700
$\dot{V}o_2$	O_2 consumption	ml/min/M^2	$\dot{V}o_2$ = CI × $a\bar{v}Do_2$ × 10	100-190
O_2 ext	O_2 extraction	%	O_2 ext = (Cao_2 − $C\bar{v}o_2$) ÷ Cao_2	20-30

H^+, nutrients, and end products of metabolism destined for excretion or recycling through distant intracellular metabolic pathways. Perfusion of the tissue must be considered from the point of view of the delivery of all requisites for cell function.

Presently, tissue perfusion cannot be measured directly. It can be approached indirectly by measuring of $\dot{V}O_2$, as well as changes in $\dot{V}O_2$ after each specific therapy, if they are given one at a time with measurements given before and after each agent. Since O_2 cannot be stored and appreciable degrees of O_2 debt cannot be accumulated for long periods of time, the rate of $\dot{V}O_2$ measured by spirometry is approximately equal to the O_2 uptake by the lung, the bulk transport of O_2 into the tissues, and the use of O_2 by the tissues. Measurement of O_2 transport variables, therefore, is the key to evaluating overall circulatory function.

Simultaneous arterial and mixed venous blood samples are collected anaerobically at the time of cardiac output estimations. Blood gases, pH, O_2 saturations, hematocrit, hemoglobin concentrations, and O_2 content are measured in samples without delay. $\dot{V}O_2$ may be measured directly by spirometry or calculated as the product of CI and the arterial-mixed venous O_2 content difference ($a\bar{v}DO_2$). $\dot{V}O_2$ should be measured directly as a check on the measurement of cardiac output by the thermodilution method. O_2 extraction rate is calculated as

$$\frac{CaO_2 - C\bar{v}O_2}{CaO_2}$$

O_2 availability (i.e., delivery of O_2 to the tissues) is measured as the product of CI and CaO_2.

Decreased $\dot{V}O_2$ indicates reduction of the overall rate of oxidative processes. In usual clinical conditions this suggests inadequate O_2 transport across the lungs; poor tissue perfusion from circulatory factors including maldistribution of flow and other microrheological alterations; or decreased metabolic rates from specific disease states such as hypothyroidism, malnutrition, vitamin deficiencies, cancericidal drugs and other metabolic poisons, hypothermia, and terminal states. Increased $\dot{V}O_2$ indicates increased tissue metabolism, which may be due to stress, sepsis, hyperthermia, posttrauma states, burns, hyperthyroidism, various drugs and anesthetics that stimulate metabolism, epinephrine, and poisons like dinitrophenol that dissociate oxidative phosphorylation. Infrequently performed measurements of $\dot{V}O_2$ give only snapshot views of the situation of the movement and may not be easily interpretable. By contrast, frequently monitored $\dot{V}O_2$ measurements taken throughout an acute illness may be exceedingly useful, especially when taken before, during, and after each therapeutic intervention given one at a time.[14] Changes in $\dot{V}O_2$ may reflect changes in tissue perfusion such as when $\dot{V}O_2$ increases after a specific agent and the therapy either improved tissue perfusion, or the agent itself stimulated increased metabolic rates.

$\dot{V}O_2$ may be greater than normal, but this does not mean that the circulation is adequate, because increased tissue requirements may be greater than the increased $\dot{V}O_2$. However, estimation of both the patient's O_2 requirements and the effect of therapy may be assessed operationally. If $\dot{V}O_2$ is greater than normal prior to therapy but does not increase after therapy, then either adequate perfusion is already present, or the $\dot{V}O_2$, though increased, is suboptimal, and the therapy is not completely ineffective. When $\dot{V}O_2$ is low before therapy and unimproved after therapy, it is concluded that the therapy was ineffective. When $\dot{V}O_2$ is low before therapy and increases afterward, then either the patient's condition spontaneously improved, or the agent may have effectively improved the circulation.[14]

REFERENCES

1. Shoemaker, W. C., and Walker, W. F.: Fluid-electrolyte therapy in acute illness, Chicago, 1970, Year Book Medical Publishers, Inc.
2. Adler, D. C., and Bryan-Brown, C. W.: Use of the axillary artery for intravascular monitoring, Crit. Care Med. **1:**148-150, 1973.
3. Skillman, J. J., Awwad, H. K., and Moore, F. D.: Plasma protein kinetics of the early transcapillary refill after hemorrhage in man, Surg. Gynecol. Obstet. **123:**983-986, 1967.
4. Wiggers, C. J.: Physiology of shock, New York, 1950, Commonwealth Fund.
5. Baek, S. M., Makabali, G. G., Bryan-Brown, C. W., Kusek, J. M., and Shoemaker, W. C.: Plasma expansion in surgical patients with high CVP, Surgery **78:**304-315, 1975.
6. Landis, E. M., and Hortenstine, J. C.: Functional significance of venous blood pressure, Physiol. Rev. **30:**1-32, Jan., 1950
7. Shoemaker, W. C.: Shock: chemistry, physiology and therapy, Springfield, Ill., 1967, Charles C Thomas, Publisher.
8. Shoemaker, W. C., Bryan-Brown, C. W., Quigley, L., Stahr, L., Elwyn, D. H., and Kark, A. E.:Body fluid shifts in depletion and post-stress states and their correction with adequate nutrition, Surg. Gynecol. Obstet. **136:**371-374, 1973.
9. Shoemaker, W. C., and Monson, D. O.: The effect of whole blood and plasma expanders on volume-flow relationships in critically ill patients, Surg. Gynecol. Obstet. **137:**453-457, 1973.
10. Davis, H. A.: Blood volume dynamics, Springfield, Ill., 1962, Charles C Thomas, Publisher.
11. Baek, S. M., Makabali, G. G., Brown, R. S., and Shoemaker, W. C.: Free-water clearance patterns as predictors and therapeutic guides in acute renal failure, Surgery **77:**632-640, 1975.
12. Vries, J. K., Becker, D. P., and Young, H. F.:A subarachnoid screw for monitoring intracranial pressure, Technical note, J. Neurosurg. **39:**416-419, 1973.
13. Swan, H. J. C., Ganz, W., Forrester, J. S., et al.: Catheterization of the heart in man with use of a flow-directed balloon-tipped catheter, N. Engl. J. Med. **283:**447-451, 1970.
14. Shoemaker, W. C.: Use of cardiorespiratory measurements to evaluate therapy and the use of therapy to evaluate pathophysiology in shock, Ann. Chir. Gynaec. Fenn. **60:**180-186, 1971.

CHAPTER 13

Data collection

Dennis M. Greenbaum

Data collection was recognized as a necessary component of intensive care as early as 1972 when Safar and Grenvik[1] reported that one responsibility of critical-care units is to develop a system of record-keeping, analysis, and review. The type of system used depends on services available in the institution. Although computers allow the largest data base and an efficient reporting mechanism,[2,3] they are not necessary for routine ICU data collection. Adequate records can be kept by a responsible member of the critical-care team without resorting to more sophisticated systems.

SELECTION OF DATA FOR COLLECTION

The most important and obvious reason to collect data is to monitor the efficacy of ICU care. Data on total ICU admissions, mortality rates, and duration of stay are examples of statistics that may reflect the quality of care.

Data collection serves other uses as well. For example, reporting of data may clarify misconceptions about ICU patients, such as the exaggerated concept of ICU mortality held by nurses and physicians. In one busy medical ICU, nurses and physicians estimated the ICU mortality rate to be about 50% before data were collected. Subsequent data showed that mortality was in fact about 25%. In the same unit, the nursing supervisor estimated the average age of ICU patients to be about 75 years. Data indicated that the average age was actually under 60 years. These two findings improved the morale of nursing staff members who previously felt that they were expending a large amount of energy for minimal returns.[4,7]

Data can also be used to test the adequacy of IC services for the needs of the institution. For example, if the ICU is too large, the occupancy rate will be low. Unfilled ICU beds are a financial burden on the institution, since a nursing staff must be provided whether or not the beds are filled. On the other hand, if the ICU is too small, it may often be overfilled. Patients will not receive adequate nursing services, since care will be diluted among a larger number of patients. In some cases, ICU candidates may even be refused admission to a critical-care area because no bed is available. The bed occupancy rate must therefore be monitored, so that a balance can be established between the number of ICU beds and the number of patients requiring intensive care. A bed occupancy rate of 75% is probably appropriate for an ICU.[5] Occasional complaints about patients being refused intensive care can be evaluated in proper perspective only when these data are available.

Sophistication of ICU services and the degree of illness can be evaluated when certain other statistics are monitored.[3,4] For example, in some units therapeutic intervention scoring systems are used. High scores suggest a greater degree of illness and/or sophistication in ICU services. Less detailed data, which indirectly reflect illness and intervention, include statistics on the number of patients receiving certain services, such as pulmonary artery catheters, transvenous pacemakers, mechanical ventilation, membrane oxygenation, or intra-aortic counterpulsation.

Data should also be kept on complications from treatment rendered in the ICU.[6] From these statistics, it may be possible to uncover a trend, suggesting a deficiency in an area of care. For example, one may find a high rate of sepsis after total parenteral nutrition, or a high rate of atelectasis after pulmonary artery catheterization. One might find an unusually high incidence of pneumonia with the use of mechanical ventilation, or of pneumothorax with the use of positive end expiratory pressure (PEEP). Correctable deficiencies in technique may be discovered that can improve intensive care.

Finally, it is important to know what type of patient is seen in the ICU. The total number of patients admitted each year, as well as a listing of diagnostic categories, is important. In one unit, members of the staff believed that more than 70% of medical ICU patients were admitted for treatment of exacerbations of chronic lung disease. However, data showed that only 8% of patients were admitted with this disorder: the discrepancy was probably due in part to the prolonged stay of these patients, which was more than double that of all ICU patients (11.7 compared to 5.6 days). The largest number of patients were admitted in cardiogenic shock.[7]

HOW TO REPORT DATA

Since statistics often disprove misconceptions about the ICU, it is important to report these data periodically to the ICU staff. All members of the ICU nursing and physician staff should receive the report. Since these data also provide information that may prevent misunderstanding regarding bed availability, use, and cost, reports[8] should be provided to the general physician staff and to the hospital administration.

At St. Vincent's Hospital and Medical Center of New York, statistics are calculated on a monthly basis and reported in an ICU newsletter (Fig. 13-1).[7] This format allows other information of interest to the ICU staff to be in-

General statistics for ICU	May, 1977	Year-to-date
ICU admissions	25	148
ICU deaths	10	40
Mortality (percent)	40	27
Postmortem permissions	3	18
Autopsy percent	30	45
Average duration of stay, all patients	3.36	5.61
Average stay, patients with COPD	7.00	13.77
Signed out AMA	0	0
Holdovers into June	5	—
Patients on mechanical ventilators	20	111
Pulmonary artery catheter (number of patients)	10	38
Readmissions*	1	13
Mean age (years)	56.1	59.5
Number of patients 70 years or under	17	98
Number of patients over 70 years	8	50
Renal transplant donors	0	0
Intra-aortic counterpulsation	0	1
Pacemakers	4	16
Bed capacity (percent)	—	71

Admissions by diagnosis	May, 1977	Year-to-date	
		Number	Survival (%)
Renal			
Peritoneal dialysis	1	9	100
Acute tubular necrosis	0	1	100
Cardiovascular			
Cardiogenic shock and preshock	6	19	42
Anaphylaxis	0	1	100
Cardiomyopathy	1	1	60
Hypovolemic shock	1	3	100
Dysrhythmia			
Acute myocardial infarction	1	8	75
Other	2	3	80

Fig. 13-1. Statistics and other information are reported monthly in medical ICU newsletter.

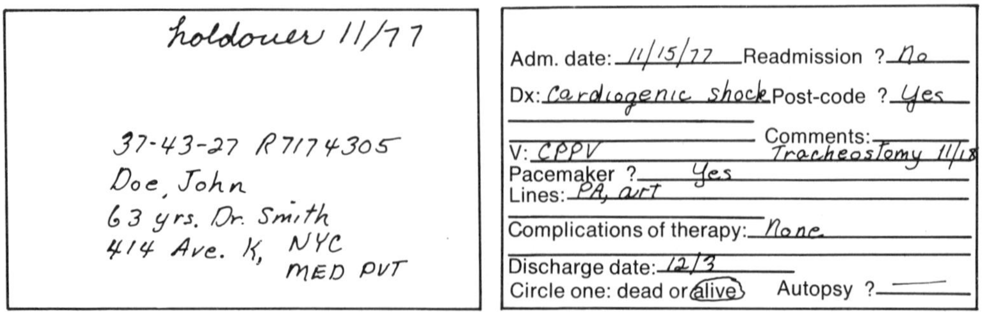

holdover 11/77

37-43-27 R7174305
Doe, John
63 yrs. Dr. Smith
414 Ave. K, NYC
MED PVT

Adm. date: _11/15/77_ Readmission ? _No_
Dx: _Cardiogenic shock_ Post-code ? _Yes_
Comments: _Tracheostomy 11/18_
V: _CPPV_
Pacemaker ? _Yes_
Lines: _PA, art_
Complications of therapy: _None_
Discharge date: _12/3_
Circle one: dead or (alive)   Autopsy ? _____

Fig. 13-2. Information card on which individual data are collected. Left, front of card and right, back of card.

Month _____		
Year _____		

General statistics	_____	Year-to-Date
ICU admissions	_____	_____
ICU deaths	_____	_____
Mortality (percent)	_____	_____
Postmortem permissions	_____	_____
Autopsy percent	_____	_____
Average duration of stay, all patients	_____	_____
Average stay, patients with COPD	_____	_____
Signed out AMA	_____	_____
Holdovers into _____	_____	_____
Patients on mechanical ventilators	_____	_____
Pulmonary artery catheters (no. of patients)	_____	_____
Readmissions	_____	_____
Mean age (years)	_____	_____
Number of patients 70 years or under	_____	_____
Number of patients over 70 years	_____	_____
Renal transplant donors	_____	_____
Intra-aortic counterpulsation	_____	_____
Pacemakers	_____	_____
Bed capacity (percent)	_____	_____
_____	_____	_____
_____	_____	_____
_____	_____	_____

Admissions by diagnosis	_____		
		Number	Survival (%)
Renal			
Peritoneal dialysis			
Acute tubular necrosis	_____	___	___
Postoperative	_____	___	___
Myoglobinuria	_____	___	___
Other	_____	___	___
_____	_____	___	___
_____	_____	___	___
_____	_____	___	___
Cardiovascular			
Cardiogenic shock and preshock	_____	___	___
Anaphylaxis	_____	___	___
Cardiomyopathy	_____	___	___
Hypovolemic shock	_____	___	___

Fig. 13-3. Front page of worksheet. Data from all individual cards collected each month are pooled in preparation for final report.

cluded, such as new equipment acquisitions, research grant approvals, and publications.

HOW TO COLLECT DATA

The simplest way to collect data is on 3- × 5-inch index cards, with entries selected so that information from the cards can be incorporated directly into the monthly report. Information is transferred from each case (Fig. 13-2) to a worksheet (Fig. 13-3). When this has been done for all cards prepared that month, the information is typed into the final report.

SUMMARY

Data collection is important for monitoring ICU activity. The statistics monitored depend on the specialization of the unit and the sophistication of data collection in the institution. Reporting accurate data can reverse misconceptions about the care provided in the ICU, and it can verify the ability of the unit to handle the number of ICU patients generated at the institution. Data collected should be reported to all professionals having contact with the ICU patients and also to hospital administrators.

REFERENCES

1. Safar, P., and Grenvik, A.: Guidelines for organization of critical care units, J.A.M.A. **222:**1532-1535, 1972.
2. Augenstein, J. S., Williams, W. H., Shapiro, E., Kaiser, G. A., Ferrero, F. A., Fried, A., Civetta, J. M., Hosek, R., and Shea, S.: A computer-based patient record system, Sixth Annual Scientific and Educational Symposium Abstracts, New York, 1977, Society of Critical Care Medicine, p. 64.
3. Kusek, J. M., Shabot, M. M., and Shoemaker, W. C.: Application of an automatic data acquisition and outcome prediction system as an index of severity to titrate therapy in critically ill surgical patients, Sixth Annual Scientific and Educational Symposium Abstracts, New York, 1977, Society of Critical Care Medicine, p. 71.
4. Kinney, J. M.: Design of the intensive care unit. In Berk, J. L., Sampliner, J. E., Artz, J. S., Vinocur, B., et al.: Handbook of critical care, Boston, 1976, Little, Brown & Co., pp. 3-20.
5. Safar, P., and Grenvik, A.: Organization and physician education in critical care medicine, Anesthesiology 47(2):82-95, 1977.
6. Zwillich, C. W., Pierson, D. J., Creagh, C. E., Sutton, F. D., Schatz, E., and Petty, T. L.: Complications of assisted ventilation: a prospective study of 354 consecutive episodes, Am. J. Med. **57:**161-170, 1974.
7. Greenbaum, D. M.:Medical ICU newsletter, New York, 1977, St. Vincent's Hospital and Medical Center of New York.
8. Cullen, D. J., Ferrara, L. C., Briggs, B. A., Walker, P. F., and Gilbert, J.:Survival, hospitalization charges and follow-up results in critically ill patients. N. Engl. J. Med. **294:**982-987, 1976.

CHAPTER 14

Critical-care problems in a developing country

Neil M. Goodwin

It was not fortuitous that intensive care and critical-care medicine first reached a high degree of sophistication in Scandinavia and the United States, because these countries have the highest standards of living and health care. Throughout the underdeveloped areas of the world, even today, poverty and ignorance combine to produce disease patterns that have not been seen in the United States for more than a century. Malnutrition, tuberculosis, and bilharziasis are all too often regarded as part of everyday existence. Urgent requirements of the local hospital are often running water and sanitary drainage, rather than for mass spectrometry in the ICU. The training of medical practitioners now occurs in many university centers throughout the tropics, and partly as a result of the two-way exchange of staff with old established centers of learning, the most highly developed critical-care techniques may today be seen side by side with traditional herbalism and even witchcraft.

It is important to appreciate that the traditions and thought processes of many races are entirely unlike those of the European or North American, and the inherited attitudes of the patient may make modern medicine unacceptable or of only partial value. To many people disease and trauma are merely manifestations of the presence of evil spirits, caused by spells that have been cast by wizards, or failure of the individual to honor ancestral spirits. In southern Africa the sick person will by tradition present himself to a "divine" or seer who, by casting the bones or by some similar device, will make a diagnosis.

After payment of an appropriate fee, the patient is then referred to an herbalist who fulfills the role of general practitioner in tribal society. The herbalist will dispense medicines made from traditional sources such as the bark of trees, roots, snake venom, or parts of various animals. To induce symptomatic relief, painful or tender areas are often marked by multiple cutaneous scarifications. By observing these, it may be possible to read the history of a disease by examining the skin alone; an example is the enlarged tender liver of amebiasis, having pain referred to the right shoulder tip.

The European physician can be likened in many ways to the herbalist, but in the eyes of the African, falls short for asking patients what is wrong with them instead of telling them! The physician, using normal techniques for obtaining details of the illness, is liable to be misled because the answers received in a sample history-taking will almost invariably be affirmative. It is bad manners to disagree with so eminent a person as the physician! To the African, events do not just happen; there is a reason behind everything. The physician is able to heal, but cannot get to the root of the problem because, as the African sees it, the physician has no concept of spirits or the significance of spells and witchcraft. A man involved in a motor vehicle accident may survive his crushed chest and other injuries in an ICU, but the intensive therapist fails for not being able to explain why the patient happened to be in his car at the place and time of the accident.

To partially compensate for these deficiencies, it may help if the approach of the ICU specialist is modified to suit local custom. The physician should not examine the conscious patient and should certainly never ask questions; assistants have already done these chores. In addition, they will have taken parts of the patient's body (blood, urine, feces, CSF, etc.) with which to cast powerful spells. If the chief ICU witch doctor is then unable to enunciate both diagnosis and prognosis, there can be little hope of survival. When this approach is employed, it is important that attention be paid to detail. For instance, evil spirits can never be killed, they can only be driven out of the body.

Selecting and training staff members for intensive care presents ethical, as well as educational problems. The most pressing requirements in many areas are not for the sophisticated care of a few severely ill patients at high cost, but general improvement of the basic health of the population. Manpower would therefore be more gainfully employed in eradicating ignorance and prejudice, and providing information on dietary requirements, and stressing the importance of prophylaxis and early referral of the sick to qualified medical personnel. If ICUs are developed on a small scale in university centers, it may be difficult for staff members to cope with the sophistication of modern electronic and other complex machinery, particularly if they were brought up in rural surroundings where electricity is unknown. However, high standards of nursing care can be achieved and maintained by imposing a strict code of discipline based on local tribal practice.

In a developing country, as in hospitals throughout the world, the location of the ICU within an existing hospital is often a compromise. Usually it will be placed close to the operating room complex to take advantage of air-conditioning and electrical supplies. Medical gases may be in short supply, and oxygen will often have to be transported over long distances. Delivery of supplies depends on climate and road conditions. Compressed air may be obtained from a small gasoline-driven compressor to power simple pressure-cycled respirators, with oxygen enrichment taking place at a T piece close to the patient. An alternative is to run the respirator directly from an oxygen cylinder, but at a very slow rate; the patient breathes room air at his own rate through a one-way valve and thus receives intermittent mandatory ventilation.

Sophisticated volume-cycled ventilators are expensive to purchase, maintain, and run; service facilities may be entirely lacking. Mechanical or electronic devices for measuring tidal volume and minute volume tend to be fragile. Emphasis on visual monitoring of the patient's chest excursion is a more reliable, practical alternative, although a simple mechanical device such as the Bennett breath-by-breath spirometer may be a useful adjunct.

Coronary artery disease is rare in many racial groups, and coronary care units are not necessary. Continuous ECG monitoring on all ICU patients is often merely an expensive source of confusion and should only be employed when absolutely essential. Durable and reusable articles for both major and minor components are still widely used, since disposable goods are expensive, must be imported, and may be supplied irregularly. All items should be easily sterilized in chlorinated or other inexpensive antiseptic solutions or by autoclaving. Gas and radiation sterilization are logistically impractical. When possible, apparatus is allowed to lie fallow in a dry atmosphere for at least 24 hours before reuse to reduce the incidence of *Pseudomonas* contamination. Rigorous, frequent cleaning (floors, walls, beds, and other apparatus) with phenolic solutions will play a more important role in the prevention of cross-infection than gowning and other operating room-oriented clothing techniques. The latter may be indicated when patients with infectious diseases such as typhoid must be cared for in the ICU because of lack of other adequate isolation facilities.

Relatives and friends visiting the unit or its environs must be rigorously controlled. With the extended family systems that pertain in many parts of the world, the immediate relations may run into many tens or even hundreds.

Witch doctors may be brought in on occasion in much the same way clergymen visit in other areas. However, we have experienced rapid deterioration of patients after such visits because of clandestine administration of herbal potions, many of which are markedly nephrotoxic and hepatotoxic.

The type of patient admitted to the African ICU tends to be very different from that in Scandinavia, for example. Geriatric patients are virtually nonexistent because priority must be given to young breadwinners. Trauma from tractor and other motor vehicle accidents is common, but many more cases will be the result of personal collisions. Penetrating knife wounds of the abdomen are often seen in hospitals many days after they were inflicted, only after unsuccessful treatment by an herbalist. The mortality from septic shock in these cases is distressingly high, even when all the known modern medical facilities are used. In contrast, septic shock from pelvic infection, usually subsequent to abortion, has a relatively low mortality rate, particularly if a total hysterectomy is performed. Death in these latter cases is usually associated with hepato-renal failure occasioned by the herbal abortifacient. It must be realized, however, that in many primitive societies a woman who cannot bear children can never marry or must be divorced and that any person who is permanently crippled, either mentally or physically, will be an added burden on a family who may already be close to starvation.

The psychological problems of the ICU patient who has previously lived in a rural area and has never seen a city, let alone a ventilator, are difficult for a western-trained physician to appreciate. Heavy sedation throughout the stay is essential, as is constant reassurance in the patient's own dialect. Many such persons find that the absence of oral food intake is almost unbearable, and the sight of a patient being ventilated through an oral endotracheal tube who happily swallows a liter of cocoa is not easily forgotten.

Despite early reports to the contrary, posttraumatic hypoxia occurs as frequently in black patients as white, but its detection may be hampered by lack of blood gas analysis facilities and by the difficulties of detecting cyanosis in those with heavily pigmented skin. An exceptionally high incidence of interstitial pulmonary edema is seen in severely shocked patients in some areas. This is partly because of a low serum albumin level, since reversal of normal albumin/globulin ratio is commonplace in many underdeveloped countries.

Much of the population lives in remote areas and travels great distances to obtain any form of medical treatment, let alone such specialties as intensive care. This, coupled with local customs and laws, leads to frequent problems over operative consent. In Zululand, all women are permanent minors and may not give consent for an operation on their own person let alone for their husband! Fortunately, litigation for imagined or even genuine malpractice is rare outside of major industrialized countries.

Many of the disease processes seen in underdeveloped areas provide remarkable material for research that is not available elsewhere. However, sophisticated investigation can seldom be undertaken because of staff and financial restrictions. Even simple follow-up of patients who have been treated and returned home presents almost insurmountable problems.

The explosive increase in foreign travel that has been seen over the past two decades has led to the frequent appearance of tropical diseases in the temperate zones. Some of these patients will be so severely ill as to require admission to an ICU, thus consideration of the following conditions may be valuable.

TYPHOID

Antonius Musa, a Roman physician, became wealthy and famous by treating the Emperor Augustus with cold baths when he fell ill with typhoid. Today typhoid is still endemic in many parts of the world, and visitors are by no means completely protected by the typhoid and paratyphoid (TAB) vaccine. After a variable onset, one or multiple intestinal perforations may appear in the patient. In many countries all perforations are considered to be caused by this bacillus until proven otherwise. This is particularly true during the rainy season, when increased contamination of domestic water sources occurs from flooding. Patients with typhoid are frequently in extremis postoperatively and require intensive care. Typhoid of this severity is a total body disease. Besides peritonitis, the patient may also have one or more of the following: impaired renal function, meningitis, fatty changes in the myocardium, and peripheral thrombophlebitis with frequent pulmonary embolism. Typhoid bronchitis is common, and lobar pneumonia is frequent. There is usually a marked neutropenia. Diagnosis is confirmed by positive blood culture, and specific therapy is still based on 1 g of chloramphenicol every 6 hours for 3 days, after which the dose is reduced to 500 mg every 6 hours for an additional 12 days. Amoxicillin and cotrimoxazole are also valuable, particularly since chloramphenicol-resistant *Salmonella* species are becoming more frequent. The differential diagnosis is not always clear cut; malaria in particular may occur concurrently. When in doubt, it is expedient to protect the patient by also administering chloroquine.

AMEBIASIS

Amebiasis is the state of an individual who harbors *Entamoeba histolytica*. The mode of presentation varies extremely, and in many persons this protozoan is a commensal parasite. Although this infection is often considered a tropical disease, its distribution is worldwide, and it has been estimated that 5% of the untraveled population in the United States is infected.

The commonest symptom is that of dysentery with variable amounts of blood and mucus. Unlike bacillary dysentery, constitutional symptoms are usually slight or absent. Positive diagnosis is by identification of the hematophagous trophozoites of *E. histolytica* in the stool or in scrapings of a rectal ulcer. Occasionally the disease is severe; the patient may have pyrexia, dehydration, and abdominal pain. The passage of fifteen or more bloody stools a day may lead to circulatory collapse and gross electrolyte disturbances, particularly hypokalemia. These patients are prone to late perforation with peritonitis and massive intestinal hemorrhage. Fulminating amebic colitis that has not responded to drug therapy is now treated by radical surgery in those hospitals in which suitable postoperative intensive care is available.

Medical therapy based on emetine, chloroquine, and tetracycline has now been revolutionized by the use of metronidazole given in doses of 800 mg every 8 hours for 5 to 10 days. Patients unable to take oral medication may benefit from suppositories or, more likely, the intravenous infusion of 500 mg of metronidazole every 8 hours.

Hepatic amebiasis with liver abscesses containing the characteristic "anchovy pus" is found more frequently in men than women. The cardinal symptom is pain over the liver and lower right chest, which may be referred to the right shoulder. Left-side symptoms are rare, as is jaundice. Amebiasic liver abscess may extend to, or rupture into, any contiguous organ. Secondary bacillary infection may occur, particularly after therapeutic or diagnostic aspiration. Hepatic amebiasis is best controlled by metronidazole, and it should be noted that tetracycline is ineffective in this form of disease.

WORM INFECTIONS

Worm infections are extremely common in developing areas of the world, yet they cause surprisingly few symptoms in the host. A heavy *Ascaris* infection may cause intestinal obstruction and jaundice due to blocking of the common bile duct. Migrating ascarides have been known to block endotracheal tubes during anesthesia and also in the ICU. Hookworms may be a cause of iron deficiency anemia, whereas a *Trichuris* infection may cause sudden death from myocardial damage by migrating larvae. Treating the majority of worm infections has been simplified by the introduction of mebendezole, which is effective even against tapeworms. Treatment is usually delayed in the critically ill patient because the sudden death of massive quantities of parasites may cause intestinal problems with colic, obstruction, and uncontrollable diarrhea.

CHRONIC DIARRHEA

Aztec two-step, Basra belly, Casablanca crud, Delhi belly, Hong Kong dog, Montezuma's revenge, Poona poohs, Simla trots, and San Franciscitis are names used by travelers to describe their most common problem—diarrhea. Many cases will be due to simple changes in water, climate, altitude, alcoholic excess, or highly spiced foods. If symptoms persist, it may be helpful to consider the following:

Infective diseases
1. Parasitic—amebiasis, bilharziasis, balantidiasis, hookworm, giardiasis, roundworm, tapeworm, malaria, trypanosomiasis
2. Nonparasitic—bacillary dysentery, salmonellosis, tuberculosis

Noninfective diseases
1. Pancreatic steatorrhea
2. Pellagra
3. Small bowel lesions such as tropical sprue, malabsorption syndrome, lymphoma, sarcoidosis
4. Granulomatous disease of colon and rectum
5. Diverticulitis and neoplasm

TETANUS

A high incidence of adult tetanus occurs in many rural communities in which effective immunization has not been carried out. In southern Africa, the extremely high incidence of neonatal tetanus is due to the traditional practice of daubing the infant's umbilicus with a mixture of mud and animal dung.

Diagnosis can usually be made on clinical grounds, although rapid onset with severe opisthotonus may make for confusion with meningitis. The site of entry must be diligently sought and surgically drained, since this will have a profound effect on the prognosis. In some patients the wound may be difficult to find; even small splinters under the toenails and fissures in the soles of the feet must be sought.

Active immunization with a toxoid does not absolutely preclude the development of tetanus, but will usually lead to a reduction in the severity of the illness. Equine antiserum is now little used. Since the efficacy of the human antiserum is doubtful, it is seldom advocated except early in high-risk patients, particularly those with burns. Prophylaxis in susceptible wounds is by high-dose, soluble penicillin with 5 million units administered every 6 hours.

A high proportion of adult patients, particularly those with long incubation periods (>14 days), will recover with simple nursing care using penicillin, heavy sedation with diazepam and chlorpromazine, but without a tracheotomy or controlled ventilation. These patients will usually show improvement after 5 to 10 days, but muscle spasm may persist for many weeks.

Patients with a severe case (incubation period < 14 days) may deteriorate to the point where respiration is grossly impaired, spasms are difficult to control, and intermittent positive pressure ventilation (IPPV) for long periods is necessary. These patients may have marked cardiovascular instability, and sudden death because of ventricular fibrillation may occur unless an alpha and beta adrenergic blockade is maintained. The current practice is to treat these patients with extremely heavy sedation for a prolonged period. A successful outcome may be obtained by totally avoiding curarization and by administering diazepam (<50 mg/hr), omnopon (<20 mg/hr), and chlorpromazine (50 to 100 mg every 6 hours). Tetanus patients will often be capable of breathing spontaneously despite a dosage of more than 1 g of diazepam and 500 mg of omnopon a day, thus minimizing deaths because of ventilator failure. A postdiazepam psychosis, which may last up to a month, will usually complicate the recovery period.

Neonatal tetanus is treated according to similar principles; ventilation is usually required for 2 to 3 weeks followed by progressive weaning using intermittent mandatory ventilation (IMV) for 1 to 2 weeks. Fortunately, since these infants have normal lungs, simple pressure-cycled respirators powered by compressed air with minimal oxygen enrichment are suitable. The most frequent complication, apart from sepsis, is difficulty in tracheal decannulation. This is most simply effected by retaining the tracheotomy tube until the infant grows, which may take up to a year. The mother must be carefully instructed on how to provide care at home for the child with a tracheostomy.

MALARIA

Malaria must be suspected in all febrile illnesses in malarial areas, and all pyrexias of unknown origin in travelers and in those living near docks or international airports. All forms of human malaria are transmitted in nature by the bite of the female *Anopheles* mosquito and like typhoid, its incidence parallels the rainfall. Occasionally, infection may occur after the transfusion of blood containing the parasites.

The severity of the disease depends on the number of parasites invading red blood cells; *Plasmodium falciparum* may affect 10% of the cells. *Plasmodium vivax*, *Plasmodium malariae*, and *Plasmodium ovale* may affect 1% to 2% of the cells. Heavy infection leads to local tissue anoxia from the blocking of capillaries, which is exaggerated by anemic anoxia. A *P. falciparum* infection in nonimmune subjects carries a 10% mortality.

The incubation period varies from 7 to 28 days or longer, depending on the species and number of parasites injected. The patient complains initially of influenzal-type symptoms, and the classical periodic pyrexia may be present. The spleen is enlarged and soft. Diagnosis is confirmed by finding malaria parasites in a thick smear of peripheral blood.

Complications of malaria are numerous and may lead to the admission of the patient to the ICU. Hyperpyrexia may be associated with delirium and convulsions. Malarial shock due to blockage of capillaries in *P. falciparum* infection causes edema of the brain, lungs, liver, and other organs, leading to hypotension, collapse, and cardiac failure, especially in those with preexisting cardiac disease. Renal lesions are also common in acute *P. falciparum* infections and may lead to oliguria with acute uremia or even anuria, necessitating hemodialysis. Blackwater fever, or acute intravascular hemolysis, usually occurs only in those who have been in endemic areas for prolonged periods. It is characterized by hemoglobinemia associated with hemoglobinuria and renal failure. Hepatic enlargement and jaundice may be encountered, and rupture of the enlarged spleen in chronic untreated cases may produce an abdominal emergency. Severe diarrhea with blood in the stools may mimic typhoid or even cholera. Disturbances of coagulation mechanisms and increased endothelial permeability have been reported in extreme cases, often as a terminal event.

In the severe form of the disease, the patient should receive chloroquine in doses of 300 mg in 150 ml of 0.9% saline solution infused over 30 minutes every 8 hours for 3 doses, after which the intravenous or intramuscular route is used until the patient can take chloroquine tablets by mouth. Chloroquine resistance is a rare occurrence, especially with *P. falciparum*, which is the usual cause of the severe disease. If resistance is suspected, 500 mg of quinine intravenously may be added to the regimen up to a total adult dosage of 2 g over 24 hours. Mepacrine is only given when other drugs are not available because of its side effects. In addition, the patient will require all the usual ICU supportive measures.

Persons at risk for malarial infection should be given one of the combinations of prophylactic schizonticides approved by the World Health Organization when traveling through or working in an endemic region. These combinations include chloroquine and primaquine or chloroquine and pyrimethamine.

BILHARZIASIS

Bilharziasis (schistosomiasis) is an insidious disease that is extremely common in developing countries. The acute phase may pass unnoticed, but the complications, especially secondary infection, may be serious and necessitate major surgery.

Urinary bilharziasis, after the red flag of hematuria in the initial infection, may give no sign until a calcified bladder, ureteric deformity, or hydronephrosis become complicated by infection. The intestinal form of the disease, besides the classical dysentery, may lead to portal hypertension from pipestem cirrhosis. Invasion of the pulmonary vasculature may lead to cor pulmonale, whereas severe status asthmaticus, because of lung sensitization to the schistosomal antigen, may occur during the invasive stage of the disease. This cause for asthma should be considered if there is a history of possible schistosomal infection and a marked eosinophilia. Dramatic response to steroid administration is seen, but recurrence is common unless the underlying disease is eradicated. In current therapy, the antimonial drugs have been replaced by the lucanthones, niridazole and hycanthone, but the dosage of these drugs must be carefully controlled. Hycanthone, which is easy to administer, is hepatotoxic and should not be given to those with a history of liver disease.

HEAT DISORDERS

Heat disorders of all kinds make their appearance only when individuals are exposed suddenly to heat at levels to which they are not accustomed or to which adaptation is not possible.

Heatstroke

Heatstroke or heat hyperpyrexia is characterized by a sudden dramatic rapid rise in body temperature to 105° F (41° C) or more, associated with neurological and mental disturbances. Initial treatment consists of removing the patient to a cool site, active correction of hyperpyrexia, control of convulsions and restlessness, rehydration, treatment of circulatory collapse, and correction of metabolic acidosis. Rapid cooling may be either by evaporation with wet towels or sheets or immersion in cold water. Military patients are best soaked or sprayed with water and driven around on the back of an open truck. Patients with severe cases should be admitted to an ICU, since they often show a picture of gram-negative septicemia associated with renal failure and disseminated intravascular coagulation (DIC).

Heat exhaustion

Water–deficiency heat exhaustion occurs because of inadequate ingestion of water. The classic symptoms are extreme thirst, weariness, and oliguria;

vomiting and anorexia are also common. The treatment consists of rehydration, which can be administered intravenously if necessary.

Salt–deficiency heat exhaustion is due to loss of excessive amounts of chloride from the body by sweating. The classical manifestations are heat cramps of the limbs and abdomen.

The differential diagnosis of heat disorders may be difficult, and indeed, some degree of overlap often exists. One profound difference is in the salt content of urine, which is high in patients with water–deficiency heat exhaustion and low in patients with salt–deficiency heat exhaustion. Pyrexia is not a constant phenomenon in either salt– or water–deficiency heat exhaustion. Correct diagnosis is important, especially when using intravenous fluids, because a 5% dextrose solution is used to correct water deficiency, and saline solutions are used in salt–deficiency heat exhaustion. Chlorpromazine, which has been advocated by some authorities for treating hyperpyrexia, should be used with caution only under circulatory supervision.

KWASHIORKOR

The name kwashiorkor comes from a Ghanaian word meaning *first, second,* referring to the fact that when the second child is born, the first loses the supply of breast milk, which is often the only source of protein. Today the more descriptive term of *protein energy malnutrition* is used. Four basic features of protein energy malnutrition are edema, growth failure, psychomotor change, and wasted muscles with overlying subcutaneous fat. No laboratory tests are required for diagnosis, but the serum albumin level indicates the severity of the disease (usually below 2 g/100 ml). Treatment consists of a high-protein, high-energy diet, which is usually based on dried skim milk. However, diarrhea because of lactose intolerance is not uncommon, and the patient may require resuscitation and total parenteral nutrition or hyperalimentation. Injections of concentrates of gamma globulin have been used by some workers, since the immune response is often severely dampened. Concurrent infections such as anemia, vitamin deficiency, and hypothermia may also require treatment.

CHOICE OF ANTIBIOTICS

The high-powered salesman of antibiotics is as ubiquitous as the Coca Cola sign, and even in developing countries, the latest products of pharmaceutical research are extolled in the mail of every physician. Resistance to simple penicillin and sulfonamides is as high in remote towns as in London, Stockholm, or New York, and in the tropics streptomycin is usually reserved for its place in tuberculosis therapy. Three compounds, however, are worthy of special consideration for both general hospital and ICU use.

Tetracycline. Despite its abuse, nephrotoxicity, and inapplicability to pediatric use, tetracycline is valuable because of its spectrum of action not only against common bacteria but also for rickettsial disease, intestinal amebiasis, brucellosis, balantidiasis, tropical sprue, and possibly cholera.

Chloramphenicol. Chloramphenicol has a bad reputation in many developed countries because of the incidence of aplastic anemia and other blood dyscrasias that occur after its administration. Enormous quantities are used in tropical areas, particularly for the treatment of diarrhea, because of its spectrum of action against typhoid and other enteric fevers. Bone marrow complications are apparently rare in black races.

Metronidazole. The antimicrobial agent metronidazole has been in use for many years for the treatment of intestinal and hepatic amebiasis, giardiasis, balantidiasis, and trichomonal infections. Recently this compound has been found to have a wide range of activity against anaerobic bacteria of many types, including *Bacteroides* and tetanus. Its relatively low cost and freedom from side effects make it a valuable drug, especially as an adjunct in treating patients with septic shock of unknown origin.

SNAKE BITE

Snake bite and its treatment are probably surrounded by more folk remedies and old wives' tales than any other medical emergency. The situation is further complicated by the fact that even when a snake has apparently bitten its victim, there is no certainty that venom has been injected. Much morbidity and mortality may in fact be attributed to the therapeutic measures that have been invoked, particularly the unnecessary application of tourniquets. The majority of snakes are not poisonous to humans.

Poisonous snakes

Cobras and mambas produce a neurotoxin that may lead to death from respiratory failure. Recovery from a mamba bite has been recorded after respiratory failure for over 72 hours, during which time the patient gave every clinical sign of brain death.

Adders and vipers produce a local cytotoxin, the effects of which will be much exaggerated if it is concentrated in a small mass of tissue by the application of a tourniquet. Shock and collapse are due to loss of fluid into the affected limb. The saw-scaled viper *(Echis cavinatus)* and occasionally other bites from this group may produce DIC.

The three species of Colubridae are peculiar to southern Africa. All are docile, and bites are usually only seen in professional snake handlers. DIC develops after 48 to 72 hours.

Antiserum

Antiserum, often polyvalent, is marketed commercially in many countries. However, it must be emphasized that this is an equine serum and should not be administered unless full facilities are present for the treatment of anaphylactic reactions. Antiserum is specific for each species of snake and therefore should only be given when appropriate. The great majority of patients will recover if basic life-support measures are applied, including ventilatory support, plasma expansion, and the treatment of DIC where applicable.

Index

☐ *t* indicates information given in table.